MEASURING
the PRICES of
MEDICAL
TREATMENTS

MEASURING the PRICES of MEDICAL TREATMENTS

Jack E. Triplett
Editor

BROOKINGS INSTITUTION PRESS
Washington, D.C.

Copyright © 1999
THE BROOKINGS INSTITUTION
1775 Massachusetts Avenue, N.W., Washington, D.C. 20036
www.brookings.edu

Library of Congress Cataloging-in-Publication data

Measuring the prices of medical treatments / Jack E. Triplett,
editor.
p. cm.
Includes bibliographical references and index.
ISBN 0-8157-8344-2 (cloth : alk. paper)
ISBN 0-8157-8343-4 (paper : alk. paper)
1. Medical care, Cost of—United States. 2. Outcome assessment
(Medical care)—United States. I. Triplett, Jack E.
RA410.53 .M388 1999   99-6229
338.4'33621'0973—dc21   CIP

9 8 7 6 5 4 3 2 1

The paper used in this publication meets minimum requirements of the
American National Standard for Information Sciences—Permanence of Paper
for Printed Library Materials: ANSI Z39.48-1984.

Typeset in Times

Composition by Northeastern Graphic Services
Hackensack, New Jersey

Printed by R. R. Donnelley and Sons
Harrisonburg, Virginia

℔ THE BROOKINGS INSTITUTION

THE BROOKINGS INSTITUTION is an independent organization devoted to nonpartisan research, education, and publication in economics, government, foreign policy, and the social sciences generally. Its principal purposes are to aid in the development of sound public policies and to promote public understanding of issues of national importance.

The Institution was founded on December 8, 1927, to merge the activities of the Institute for Government Research, founded in 1916, the Institute of Economics, founded in 1922, and the Robert Brookings Graduate School of Economics and Government, founded in 1924.

The Board of Trustees is responsible for the general administration of the Institution, while the immediate direction of the policies, program, and staff is vested in the President, assisted by an advisory committee of the officers and staff. The by-laws of the Institution state: It is the function of the Trustees to make possible the conduct of scientific research, and publication, under the most favorable conditions, and to safeguard the independence of the research staff in pursuit of their studies and in the publication of the result of such studies. It is not a part of their function to determine, control, or influence the conduct of particular investigations or the conclusions reached.

The President bears final responsibility for the decision to publish a manuscript as a Brookings book. In reaching his judgment on competence, accuracy, and objectivity of each study, the President is advised by the director of the appropriate research program and weighs the views of a panel of expert outside readers who report to him in confidence on the quality of the work. Publication of a work signifies that it is deemed a competent treatment worthy of public consideration but does not imply endorsement of conclusions or recommendations.

The Institution maintains its position of neutrality on issues of public policy in order to safeguard the intellectual freedom of the staff. Hence interpretations or conclusions in Brookings publications should be understood to be solely those of the authors and should not be attributed to the Institution, to its trustees, officers, or other staff members, or to the organizations that support its research.

Foreword

ECONOMIC STATISTICS can provide a picture of our economy—where it is and where it has been. But perhaps the metaphor is better extended to a video recording, because the economy is always changing, and we most want to know about the movements within that picture (the rate of inflation, the rate of economic growth).

Economists know that making this particular video is harder than it looks. Measuring the economy well means incorporating all the new products and new services and technological changes that affect the way goods and services are produced and brought to final consumers. The economic picture requires not just enumerating and keeping track of the bewildering number of new and improved products, new methods of delivery, and so forth, but also putting a value on them. That is the hard part. What is it worth, for example, to have mobile telephones compared with stationary ones? What is the value of this technological advance?

No part of the economy poses more of these valuation problems than the medical care sector. What is the rate of medical inflation? The change in output of the medical care sector? The productivity of the resources—nearly one-seventh of GDP—put into medical care? The effect of increased consumption of medical services on health? Answering those important questions, even approximately well, requires putting a value on changes in medical treatments.

For example, medical researchers have documented the sharp decline in mortality from heart attacks. Although there are a number of causes, improved methods for treating heart attacks have contributed greatly to the decline in mortality. But, generally, improved treatments cost more than older ones. When medical expenditures increase because of improved and more expensive treatments, how much of this rise (if any) is medical inflation? And how much is the value of improved medical treatments? What are improved treatments worth? Sometimes it is thought inappropriate to ask that question of medical care, but medical output, medical inflation, and medical productivity statistics all require that a value be placed on improvements in medical treatments.

Quite recently new techniques for measuring the prices of medical treatments have been developed. This research still covers only a small proportion of medical care expenditures, but its results are provocative. They suggest that medical care inflation is not nearly so severe as sometimes thought, provided appropriate allowances are made in economic statistics for the value of improvements in medical treatments.

In November 1997 the Brookings Institution and the American Enterprise Institute for Public Policy Research held a conference on many of these issues raised in the debate over how we measure the prices of medical treatments. This volume is one of the results of that meeting, which was supported by Eli Lilly and Company and Sidney Taurel, chairman, president and chief executive officer, whose support is gratefully acknowledged.

Among the contributions that made the conference a success, Robert B. Helms, director of Health Policy Studies at AEI, and his assistant, Sharon Utz, are foremost. Valuable advice and assistance were rendered by Thomas W. Croghan, Ann Nobles, and Douglas Cocks of Lilly. At the Brookings Institution Press, Marian Schwartz edited the manuscript, Carlotta Ribar proofread the final pages, and Julia Petrakis provided an index. Helen Kim and Jane Kim provided research assistance to Jack Triplett.

The views expressed here are those of the authors and should not be ascribed to the institutions that supported this work, or to the trustees, officers, or staff members of the Brookings Institution.

MICHAEL H. ARMACOST
President

June 1999
Washington, D.C.

Contents

MEASURING
the PRICES of
MEDICAL
TREATMENTS

1

Introduction:
New Developments in
Measuring Medical Care

Jack E. Triplett and Ernst R. Berndt

HOW SERIOUS IS medical care inflation in the United
States? Between 1986 and 1996 the medical care
component of the consumer price index (CPI) rose 6.5 percent per year,
which far exceeds the 3.6 percent annual increase in the overall CPI
during this period.

However, constructing accurate price indexes for medical markets is
especially difficult, and many economists believe that economic statistics
do not accurately measure medical care price changes. Contrary to the
usual presumption of runaway medical inflation, some very recent research, reported in this volume, suggests that prices for at least some
medical care interventions are not rising rapidly and may even be falling.

Understanding medical care inflation is important for topics such as
policy toward medical care cost containment. If medical care inflation
is not the driving force behind the run-up in medical care costs, as the
studies included in this volume suggest, then medical care costs are
being driven by real changes in the quantity of care. This finding, if
confirmed by studies on other medical procedures, suggests that health
care cost containment may have social costs—curtailment of health care
that has real impacts on health—that are more severe than are generally
recognized.

Medical care price indexes not only indicate the rate of medical care
inflation, they also affect other economic statistics on medical care. For
example, measures of the output of the medical care sector and of the
consumption of medical care in national accounts use medical care price
indexes as deflators, as explained in a subsequent section. Errors in the

deflators create parallel errors in the measures of medical care output and of consumption. Thus our understanding of the most important economic trends in the medical care sector is vitally dependent on accurate medical care price measures.

This volume brings together state-of-the-art methodological and empirical work on the measurement of medical outcomes and prices. The chapters in it were originally presented as papers at a conference that was jointly sponsored by the Brookings Institution and the American Enterprise Institute for Public Policy.

Background

Information on aggregate U.S. medical care expenditures appears in the National Income and Product Accounts (NIPA) of the Bureau of Economic Analysis (BEA) and in the National Health Accounts (NHA) of the Health Care Financing Administration (HCFA). The latter provide the frequently cited statistic that the United States spends one-seventh of gross domestic product on medical care, the highest percentage in the world.

Medical care expenditures, of course, are the product of price and quantity. In national accounting language, the quantity of medical care is called "real" medical care expenditures. We can interpret real medical care expenditures as the output of the medical care sector and as the consumption of medical care by the U.S. population.

In national accounts, one normally estimates real medical care expenditures by removing estimated medical inflation from the increase in actual expenditures on medical care. This process is known as "deflation." Effectively, any increase in medical care expenditures that is *not* inflation is an increase in the quantity of health care, where the quantity, in this way of looking at it, includes both changes in the number of treatments and changes in the quality or effectiveness of treatments.

With the deflation methodology, any error in the price indexes that measure medical inflation creates an equal error of opposite sign in the real expenditure, or quantity, data. Thus accurate price indexes for medical care are important both because they measure medical care inflation and because they are used to measure medical care real expenditures.

Historically, the major source of information on U.S. medical care inflation was the medical care component of the consumer price index published by the Bureau of Labor Statistics (BLS). Health economists have long suspected that the CPI medical care price indexes have errors, and most have believed that they rise too rapidly. If measured medical price inflation has been overstated, then the NIPA and the NHA have understated improvement in the quantity of medical care. That problem has motivated research on medical care price indexes.

The CPI is designed to answer the question: How much out-of-pocket expenditures would be necessary in the current year to buy the basket of goods and services that was bought in the base year?[1] Medical care goods and services are included in the CPI basket.

However, on the CPI's definition, only those medical care commodities purchased directly by households, and only the proportion of them financed by out-of-pocket expenditures, are within the scope of the index. For this reason, the items chosen for CPI pricing were weighted toward those that are more frequently purchased from out-of-pocket expenditures.

For many purposes, economists and health policy analysts wanted to know—not the increase in prices for the consumer out-of-pocket portion of medical expenses, which corresponded to the CPI concept—but the price change for the full medical care sector. When they used the CPI as an indicator of price change for the whole medical care sector, they found it had a persistent shortcoming: Some expenditures, such as payments by employer-provided medical insurance, were outside the scope of the CPI definition of consumption. Additionally, the CPI did not collect discounts that third-party payers, such as insurance companies, obtained from medical care providers.

Another problem arose because for the old CPI (before 1997) the Bureau of Labor Statistics chose a sample of medical care charges—a visit to a doctor's office, administration of a standardized medicine (such as an influenza shot), the daily room rate in a hospital, and so forth. When the CPI medical care component was constructed from the price of a hospital room rate, one expects a substantial bias relative to the cost of treating a disease because the average number of days in the hospital for a specified disease is declining. For example, the average length of stay for heart attack patients has fallen from fifteen days in 1975 to eight days in 1995,[2] and the average hospital stay for cataract surgery has

---

1. The price index is formed from a ratio that takes as the numerator the hypothetical expenditure level that is the answer to this question and as the denominator the actual expenditures in the base year. The price index is usually expressed with the base year set equal to 100. In concept, the CPI is a fixed weight approximation to a cost-of-living index, where the cost-of-living index measures the cost in the current period of the standard of living achieved in the base period.

2. Heidenreich and McClellan (1998).

fallen from seven days in 1952 to zero currently because the surgery has become an outpatient procedure.[3] Similarly, collecting the price for a doctor's office visit would, one expects, yield a substantially biased price index when new technology greatly expands what the doctor can do during that visit.

As Dennis Fixler points out (see his comments to chapters 2 and 3), the Bureau of Labor Statistics has recently addressed both these problems. Beginning in 1992, a new series of industry medical care price indexes was introduced into the producer price index (PPI). The PPIs for hospitals and for physicians' offices are based on charges to all payers, not just consumer out-of-pocket expenditures.

Additionally, the Bureau of Labor Statistics adopted a new, improved methodology for pricing medical care for the PPI. In the new methodology, the BLS obtains prices for a sample of specified treatments for particular diseases, rather than for a day in the hospital. The improved pricing methodology was extended to the CPI in 1997. Economists agree that this new methodology is a great improvement compared with the old one.

In its new price indexes the BLS has not, however, fully solved the difficult problem of allowing for quality change in medical treatments—changing medical technology that results in improved medical outcomes. This problem motivates most of the research summarized in this volume.

An additional part of the health measurement problem concerns price indexes for prescription pharmaceuticals. Here, again, research suggests that price indexes have in the past overstated the increase in medical price inflation.

Researchers, primarily those at the National Bureau of Economic Research (NBER), undertook several detailed evaluations and critiques of the BLS's CPI and PPI prescription drug components. Zvi Griliches and Iain Cockburn pointed out that the BLS former treatment of generic drugs—as new goods, not directly comparable to their originator branded predecessors—resulted in overstated price inflation because no price decreases were recorded in the indexes when new, cheaper generics became available.[4] Ernst Berndt, Zvi Griliches, and Joshua Rosett also presented evidence suggesting that the PPI program oversampled middle- and older-aged drugs and undersampled newer pharmaceutical products.[5] Because price increases were larger for older than for younger

3. Shapiro and Wilcox (1996).
4. Griliches and Cockburn (1994).
5. Berndt, Griliches, and Rosett (1993).

drugs, those results implied that growth in producer price indexes for pharmaceuticals overstated true price growth. Studies by IMS, a data firm specializing in pharmaceuticals, and by BLS researchers corroborated the empirical findings of Berndt, Griliches, and Rosett.[6]

Partly in response to that set of research findings, the BLS implemented changes in both its CPI and PPI prescription drug components. The CPI now treats a branded drug and its generic equivalent as the same product rather than as different products—the previous price index treatment. With the new methodology, the introduction of a generic causes the price index to fall, as it should.[7]

The BLS's prescription drug PPI program has implemented two sets of changes—one involving generics and the other supplementary sampling to bring newly introduced pharmaceuticals into the sample more quickly. Douglas Kanoza and Gregory Kelly outlined those changes.[8] Their impact has been substantial. As Kelly has discussed, the combined impact of changing the treatment of generics and supplementary sampling of newer drugs has reduced measured inflation in the prescription drug PPI from 4.1 percent (under older procedures) to 3.3 percent (using new procedures) between January 1996 and March 1997.

What Do We Want in Economic Statistics on Medical Care? And Why Do We Want It?

Most economists, public policy analysts, and health industry professionals want to separate spending increases on health care into price increases and quantity increases. But some conference participants questioned the premise: Why do we want measures of price change for medical care? And why do we need to adjust the price indexes for the value of improved medical technology? Charles Phelps (comments to chapters 2 and 3) and Mark Pauly (chapter 6) address the question, but perhaps it deserves a lengthier and more explicit discussion.

Phelps and Pauly give compatible answers. Pauly contends: "A price index should tell us how much better or worse off price changes make a particular set of consumers. Slightly more formally, if the expenditure on a particular good or basket of goods changes, a price index measures the

6. Ristow (1996); Kanoza (1996); Kelly (1997).

7. U.S. Department of Labor, Bureau of Labor Statistics (undated) provides a more detailed description of the new BLS procedures involving the CPI for prescription drugs.

8. Kanoza (1996); Kelly (1997).

amount of additional income needed to be provided to the consumer (for price increases) or taken away from the consumer (for price decreases) to leave him or her as well off as before a change."

In addition, both scholars gave the same reason for wanting to treat quality improvements in health care as if they were increases in the quantity of care. According to Pauly: "It is obvious that when quality changes, the measure of the change in total expenditure needs to be adjusted to account for the quality change. . . . One reason why an improved price index for medical services . . . is an issue is precisely because we have strong reasons to believe that the quality of those services has been changing over time."

The Phelps-Pauly way of looking at the problem of measuring medical care prices is not so different from the way one measures economic activity in the rest of the economy. Compilers of national health accounts and the national income and product accounts always produce measures of "real" spending, in which increased quantities are separated from price movements (inflation).[9] Increased quantities are associated with in- creased consumption. Other things equal, increasing per capita consump- tion translates into increased economic welfare of consumers.

Yet one suspects that saying "we do it for the other parts of the economy" may not convince everyone. One stereotype about health has increased medical spending driven by medical care inflation. Much of the discussion surrounding the Clinton administration's health care reform initiative repeated that idea: Health care prices were rising too rapidly, many health care policy analysts contended, and the policy problem was to contain those "out-of-control" price increases. Indeed, as Phelps re- marked, rapid health care inflation has been "the fundamental premise of health care policy over the past decades."

But medical care has another stereotype: The quantities produced and consumed are excessive. Observers often allege that the United States has too many high-tech medical procedures, overprescription of pharma- ceuticals, excessive care of various types, too much "defensive" medicine, and so forth. One suspects that the policy analysts who are unconvinced about the need for measuring the quality of medical care would say, "So you have shown me that some of what I thought was medical price inflation is actually increased medical quantities; but I don't care, because the quantities are too great anyway." They are contending, in effect, that

9. See Levit and others (1996) for the health accounts and U.S. Department of Commerce (1985) for the national income and product accounts.

medical care is different: Increased consumption of apples and oranges may represent increased welfare for consumers, but increased consumption of medical care does not necessarily increase welfare.

Indeed, Pauly asserts, "virtually the entire American health care policy analysis in the past thirty years has been based on the view that the medical market did not function like ordinary markets. . . . Whether the cause was health insurance, consumer ignorance and consequent demand inducement, or a postulated 'technological imperative,' the effect was hypothesized to be the same: U.S. medical care sector has fostered some changes in technology whose value has fallen far short of their cost."

Researchers have also confronted that challenge. One does not want an accurate price index for medical care solely to determine that part of medical expenditure increases were driven by increased quantities of medical procedures. Indeed, we knew that, even without a price index.

The underlying issue, as several of the studies stated explicitly, is whether or not the increased use of medical procedures improves patient outcomes. If new medical technologies have a value that falls short of their cost, as is sometimes asserted, then price indexes that accurately account for the value of quality change in health care will rise; additionally, real health care expenditures (or quantity) will grow less rapidly than actual expenditures.

Conversely, if the value of new technology exceeds its cost, the price indexes will fall, even if medical expenditures are rising; and measures of real medical expenditures will rise even more rapidly. For example, David Cutler, Mark McClellan, and Joseph Newhouse (chapter 2) state: "We define the change in the cost-of-living index as the increased spending on medical care over time less the additional value of that care. If medical care increases in cost without much improvement in health, that would be an increase in the cost of living. If medical care increases in cost but the value of that care rises over time, the cost-of-living index would be falling."

To estimate such "quality-adjusted" price indexes, one needs to be able to connect measures of medical outcomes with expenditures on medical treatments. The crucial measurement issue, then, is the valuation of medical care improvements. Obtaining accurate information on the relations among price change, quantity change, changes in medical outcomes, and expenditure change is the real objective of improved economic statistics on medical care treatments.

Quantitative measures of medical outcomes thus play an essential role in improving economic measurement of the medical sector. Cutler, McClellan, and Newhouse (chapter 2), Richard Frank, Ernst Berndt, and

Susan Busch (chapter 3), Pauly (chapter 6), and also Joel Hay and Winnie
Yu (chapter 5), who call attention to the lack of a sufficient quantity of
medical outcome information, emphasize the importance of that role.
Jack Triplett (chapter 7) points out that the absence of medical outcome
measures in the past has left the nation's economic statistics on medical
care inadequate and frequently criticized.[10] John Eisenberg (chapter 8)
points the way to government-sponsored improvements in information
on medical outcomes that could in principle be used to make economic
statistics on health care better reflect the contribution of medical care to
improvements in health.

The objection that medical quantities may be excessive and may not
be good indicators of welfare has some validity as a general statement of
a problem. Medical care differs in some ways from many other consumption goods and services (although not necessarily from all of them), in the
sense that there is great concern within the medical profession and the
policymaking community about the relative efficacy and cost-effectiveness of some forms of medical treatment. But economists have not ignored that problem. Far from it. One of the recurring themes in the
studies reviewed here was the need—for economic measurement as well
as for other purposes—of exactly the measures of medical outcome that
would tell us whether increased quantities of medical care really do
improve the welfare of medical care recipients.

A panel discussion involving John Eisenberg, Willard Manning, David
Meltzer, and Burton Weisbrod (chapter 8) explores some deeper issues
that are closer to the frontiers of economic understanding. Manning and
Meltzer, as well as Weisbrod, emphasize that a price index is closely
related to a measure of economic welfare, although that is sometimes not
recognized in the pragmatic use of the statistics that government agencies
produce. Except for very narrowly specified purposes, however, we do not
ultimately want to know about the price change for a particular treatment.
Pricing treatments is, as Manning (chapter 8) puts it, a move in the right
direction because it brings us closer to what is ultimately wanted. Ideally,
economists want to measure the cost of producing increased survival and
improved quality of life. We ultimately want to know, as Meltzer (chapter
8) notes, whether expenditures on health care are worth it. That requires
us to put a value on health care and on improving health.

The problem—and this is what makes the measurement of health care
really hard—is that knowing how to measure health in its broad dimen-

10. For an example of that criticism, see Newhouse (1989).

sion requires knowing a great deal about individuals' preferences for different health states and alternatives that might be produced for the same expenditure of medical resources. For example, measures of medical outcomes such as QALY (quality-adjusted life-years) explicitly require information about preferences among different health outcomes.[11]

Manning (chapter 8) and Weisbrod (chapter 8) also address another serious omission in existing measures of the cost of health care. BLS price indexes, the national accounts as produced by the BEA, the national health accounts as produced by HCFA, and most estimates of cost-of-living indexes (such as in chapter 2), omit all nonmarket costs of illness and of receiving health care. Such nonmarket costs are outside the traditional "production boundary" of the national accounts. In Manning's example, if someone withdraws from the labor force to care for a family member (instead of continuing to work and placing the family member in a nursing home), the national accounts assume that the time devoted to such care is worth nothing. Of course, that is true of the national accounts (and CPI) treatment of all economic activities so it is not unique to the national accounts treatment of health care. But as these economists pointed out, the issue looms larger in the case of health care, because time costs are associated with the care of others and with obtaining care for oneself. Omitting those costs seems likely to bias significantly our understanding of changes in the cost, or price, of health care.

The Costs and Benefits of Intensive Treatment for Cardiovascular Disease

In chapter 2, Cutler, McClellan, and Newhouse summarize a continuing research program on the treatment of heart attacks that they are conducting in collaboration with other researchers. In this research, they examined changes in the technology for treating heart attacks, estimated the impact of changes in technology and in pharmaceuticals on survival probabilities, determined the sources of increased costs for treating heart

---

11. "The QALY (quality-adjusted life-years) is a measure of health outcome that assigns to each period of time a weight, ranging from 0 to 1, corresponding to the quality of life during that period, where a weight of 1 corresponds to perfect health and a weight of 0 corresponds to a health state judged equivalent to death. The number of quality-adjusted life-years, then, represents the number of healthy years of life that are valued equivalently to the actual health outcome" [Gold and others (1996), p. 29]. QALY estimates are being employed in cost-effectiveness studies on medical interventions.

Table 1-1. *Changes in U.S. Heart Attack Mortality, 1975–95*

U.S. heart attack deaths	1975	1995	Change (thousands)	Change (percent)
Total (thousands)[a]	325	218	−107	−32.9
Per 100,000 population[b]	152	83	−69	−45.5
Per 100,000 population (age-adjusted)[c]	107	44	−64	−59.2
In-hospital heart attack deaths (thousands)[d]	75	76	+1	+1.3

a. The 1975 number was calculated from the rate of heart attacks (.1524 percent), and the population (213,032,000). Source: U.S. Department of Health, Education and Welfare, National Center for Health Statistics (HEW, NCHS), 1979, *Vital Statistics of the United States, 1975: Volume II—Mortality, Part A*, Hyattsville, Md., pp. 1–7, table 1-7, and p. 6–23, table 6-2.

b. 1975 data source: HEW, NCHS, 1979, *Vital Statistics of the United States, 1975: Volume II—Mortality, Part A*. Hyattsville, Md.: National Center for Health Statistics. 1995 data source: U.S. Department of Health and Human Services, Centers for Disease Control and Prevention, and National Center for Health Statistics (HHS, CDC, and NCHS), 1997, *Monthly Vital Statistics Report* 45(11) (supplement 2) (June 12), p. 20, table 6.

c. 1975 data were age adjusted by using the method used by the National Center for Health Statistics (HHS, CDC, and NCHS, *Technical Appendix from Vital Statistics of the United States: 1994, Mortality*. Hyattsville, Md.: National Center for Health Statistics, 1994, http://www.cdc.gov/nchswww/data/techap94.pdf, pp. 28, 32). $R^* = \Sigma w_i R_i$, where R^* is the age-adjusted rate, w_i is the population weight (provided in the *Technical Appendix*) and R_i is the age-specific rate for the ith age group. The weights are based on the age structure of the U.S. population in 1940. The NCHS advised that the comparison between data before 1979 and after is not completely compatible, since the ICD-9-CM replaced the ICDA/ICD-8 in 1979, and coding changes may have occurred. 1995 data source: HHS, CDC, and NCHS, 1997, *Monthly Vital Statistics Report* 45(11) (supplement 2) (June 12), p. 20, table 6.

d. The number of in-hospital AMI deaths recorded by NCHS. 1975 source: HHS, NCHS, 1978, *Vital and Health Statistics: Inpatient Utilization of Short-Stay Hospitals by Diagnosis: United States, 1975*, series 13 (35), table R. 1995 source: HHS, NCHS, 1998, *Vital and Health Statistics: National Hospital Discharge Survey: Annual Summary, 1995*, series 13(133), p. 13, table L.

attacks, and finally proposed an answer to the question, Was the increased expenditure worth it?

Cutler and his colleagues demonstrate what economic research on medical treatments can do and provide a greater understanding of what remains to be done. Coupled with the quite different work on a different disease—mental depression—by Frank, Berndt, and Busch (chapter 3), the study provides a model that researchers could well follow to analyze other medical conditions.

The setting for the study by Cutler, McClellan, and Newhouse is the remarkable decline in the mortality implications of heart attacks. According to the National Center for Health Statistics (NCHS), the number of recorded U.S. heart attack deaths declined by about a third between

1975 and 1995 (table 1-1). Over that twenty-year period, however, the population grew and the age structure of the population shifted toward the older groups that are more vulnerable to heart attacks, so the improvement in mortality was greater than the impression conveyed by the unadjusted numbers. The NCHS calculated that the heart attack death rate declined by 45 percent between 1975 and 1995 and that the age-adjusted rate declined by nearly 60 percent.[12]

Why has the heart attack death rate declined? A heart attack is not the only outcome of heart disease, nor is it the only cause of death from heart disease. Heart attacks account for a little less than half of recorded deaths from ischemic heart disease.[13] Heart attack deaths will decline with reductions in heart disease and heart attack incidences (and also severity), which might be attributable to direct medical intervention—more aggressive treatment of high blood pressure with pharmaceuticals, for example—or to nonmedical sources, such as changes in diet or in exercise habits or less smoking. Prevention is not addressed directly in this study, which examines the treatment of heart attacks.

What happens after a victim suffers a heart attack? A heart attack, when detected, requires treatment in a hospital. The first step to treatment is therefore to get the victim to a hospital, and some die before receiving any hospital treatment; indeed, more than three-quarters of heart attack deaths occurred outside hospitals in 1975 and about 65 percent in 1995 (compare total heart attack deaths and in-hospital heart attack deaths in table 1-1).

Table 1-1 implies a substantial drop in out-of-hospital deaths from heart attacks. Between 1975 and 1995, the number of heart attack deaths occurring in hospitals was effectively unchanged when the total number of heart attack deaths declined about one-third. Most of the total two-decade decline in heart attack deaths occurred because of a sharp reduction in the number of heart attack victims who died before reaching a

12. The published NCHS rates are given in table 1-1. Regrettably, the NCHS age-adjusted rates use as weights the age structure of the United States in 1940. In 1940, ages sixty-five and over accounted for only about 7 percent of the population, so the weights used by NCHS are not close to those of either 1975 or 1995. The magnitudes of the declines reported in table 1-1 are so large that reweighting is unlikely to affect the major conclusion.

13. NCHS, *Monthly Vital Statistics Report* (June 12, 1997), table 8. In 1995, the numbers were 481,000 and 218,000, respectively, for ischemic heart disease and heart attack deaths, giving a ratio of 45 percent. Ischemic heart diseases are those that are caused by or that cause obstruction of the blood supply to the heart. Deaths from old heart attacks contribute a portion of deaths classified among non-heart attack, ischemic heart disease deaths.

hospital and, perhaps, after discharge from a hospital. The decline in out-of-hospital heart attack deaths is over 40 percent.[14]

In a review of the medical literature on heart attack treatments, Paul Heidenreich and Mark McClellan reported that existing studies of initial treatment changes (such as advanced cardiac life-support facilities in emergency vehicles) fail to explain much of the out-of-hospital death rate decline: "The actual improvements in prehospital technologies appear to account for only a modest increase in the number of [heart attack] patients reaching the hospital alive."[15] Heidenreich and McClellan also noted that changes in coding practices may account for some of the recorded decline in nonhospital heart attack deaths (because those cases are sometimes difficult to classify in the absence of an autopsy) and that reporting errors appear to be correlated with reported incidence rates. Yet the aggregate numbers indicate that nonhospital heart attack deaths have dropped substantially, and it is difficult to believe that all of that drop could result from measurement error.

Of course, a nonhospital heart attack death averted might only result in an in-hospital death. Indeed, one expects that the most severe heart attack victims, on average, are likelier to die before hospitalization. If a higher proportion of heart attack victims did reach the hospital in 1995 (as noted, it is not certain that such is the case), then those cases increase at the margin the severity of the cases the hospital must treat. Heidenreich and McClellan cited fragmentary evidence in favor of that "marginal" patient hypothesis.[16]

The actual story seems to be that the average severity of heart attack hospitalizations has declined, even if the marginal cases have increased in severity. Cutler, McClellan, and Newhouse review several measures of heart attack severity among hospital patients and conclude that "average [heart attack] case severity decreased slightly, potentially accounting for 10–20 percent of the decline in the average . . . mortality rate." Heidenreich and McClellan concluded that "the bulk of the evidence suggests that changes in the nature of [heart attacks] in hospitalized patients accounts for a significant part of the observed improvements in outcomes," particularly before 1985.[17]

---

14. The unadjusted numbers, calculated from the data in table 1-1, are 250,000 in 1975 and 142,000 in 1995. Out-of-hospital deaths from heart attacks are not published separately on an age-adjusted basis.

15. Heidenreich and McClellan (1998).

16. Ibid.

17. Ibid.

Thus something has reduced the number of heart attacks that cause death before hospitalization and presumably has also reduced the severity of cases that are hospitalized. We cannot determine at present whether the causal factors are improvements in general health of the population, changes in primary prevention methods, or something else.[18]

What has happened to heart attack victims once they reach the hospital? According to NCHS data, the actual number of in-hospital heart attack deaths has hardly changed (table 1-2). Because the population has grown, a more relevant statistic is the hospital death rate, or case fatality rate. But the aggregate NCHS data on heart attack hospitalizations, and thus also the hospital death rate, are ambiguous.

Two NCHS classifications for heart attack hospitalizations exist. "All listed" includes any hospital discharge where heart attack is mentioned among the diagnoses. "First listed" means that a heart attack was the principal condition "established after study to be chiefly responsible for occasioning the admission."[19] Constructing a consistent time series is complicated by a coding change in 1982 that transferred some 200,000 cases into the first-listed category of heart attacks.[20]

We have adjusted the published NCHS first-listed hospital discharge time series by estimating the effect of the 1982 coding change.[21] The result, shown in table 1-2, is an increase of 216,000 heart attack hospitalizations between 1975 and 1995, a little less than 40 percent.

However, Heidenreich and McClellan (1998), working with National Hospital Discharge Survey (NHDS) microdata and other longitudinal data sources, rather than published NCHS tabulations, have noted substantial increases in transfers and readmissions.[22] They adjust heart attack discharges additionally for these effects and report (table 1-2) that adjusted new heart attack discharges actually fell. There are probably inconsistencies between the number of heart attack hospitalizations computed by researchers from NCHS microdata and the total estimated from the same data by NCHS, so those inconsistencies should be kept in mind when interpreting the data in table 1-2. Nevertheless, hospital

18. Heidenreich and McClellan (1998) review evidence on changes in population risk factors.
19. U.S. Department of Health and Human Services (1995).
20. The coding change, which raised the proportion of heart attack discharges that were coded as "first-listed," was intended to correct improper coding (when a heart attack victim is hospitalized, the heart attack is seldom a secondary consideration). In 1982, the first-listed series increased by 230,000 (50 percent), the all-listed series by only 13,000. No consistent time series of heart attack hospitalizations is published by NCHS.
21. The derivation of the adjusted estimate is explained in note b of table 1-2.
22. Heidenreich and McClellan (1998).

Table 1-2. *Hospital Discharges and Fatality Rates, U.S. Heart Attacks,*
1975–95

U.S. heart attack deaths	1975	1995	Change (thousands)	Change (percent)
In-hospital heart attack deaths, by first-listed diagnosis (thousands)[a]	75	76	+1	+1.3
Hospital discharges, heart attacks, first-listed				
Adjusted for coding change (thousands)[b]	555	771	+216	+38
Adjusted for transfers, etc. (thousands)[c]	542	540	−2	−0.5
In-hospital fatality rate (percent of first-listed heart attacks)				
Adjusted for coding change[d]	13.5	9.9	−3.6	−26.7
Adjusted for transfers, etc., and also age-sex adjusted	23	14	−9	−39
30-day fatality rate (percent)[f]	27	17	−10	−36

a. The number of in-hospital AMI deaths recorded by NCHS. 1975 source: HHS, NCHS, 1978, *Vital and Health Statistics: Inpatient Utilization of Short-Stay Hospitals by Diagnosis: United States, 1975*, series 13 (35): table R. 1995 source: HHS, NCHS, 1998, *Vital and Health Statistics: National Hospital Discharge Survey: Annual Summary, 1995*, series 13(133): 13, table L.

b. In 1982, a coding change affecting first-listed heart attack diagnoses became effective. The 1981 number of first-listed heart attacks is corrected for this coding change, as follows (data come from various issues of NCHS, *Vital and Health Statistics,* series 13):

First, the average annual percentage changes of first-listed diagnoses (2.97 percent) and of all-listed diagnoses (1.57 percent) were calculated for 1975 through 1981. There is a steady upward drift, of first-listed relative to all-listed heart attack discharges, of a little over one percentage point per year. On the assumption that the same drift would be present in consistently coded series for 1981 and 1982, the difference in these two rates (1.38 percentage points) was added to the 1981–82 percent change for all-listed diagnoses; the resulting percentage change became the corrected percent change in first-listed diagnoses between 1981 and 1982. The adjusted time series of first-listed diagnoses was calculated for each preceding year (1975–81) by applying to the adjusted 1981 number the percentage changes in first-listed diagnoses from the published NCHS data. 1975 source used for calculation: HHS, 1978, *Vital and Health Statistics: Inpatient Utilization,* pp. 26, 50; tables 1 and 5. 1995 source: HHS, 1998, *Vital and Health Statistics: National Hospital Discharge,* p. 5, table B.

c. Adjusted for transfers and readmissions. Source: Heidenreich, Paul, and Mark McClellan, 1998, "Trends in Technology Use for Acute Myocardial Infarction," manuscript, table 1.

d. The 1975 and 1995 data are calculated by dividing in-hospital heart attack deaths by hospital discharges, adjusted for coding change (for example, the 1975 entry is 75 divided by 555, which equals .135.

e. Adjusted for age and gender (1975 levels), in Heidenreich and McClellan, "Trends," table 1.

f. Based on an exponential decline in daily mortality from day 7 to day 30, in Heidenreich and McClellan, "Trends," table 1.

fatality rates computed with either adjusted series fell substantially between 1975 and 1995—by at least a quarter, and perhaps by nearly 40 percent. The latter estimate contains an additional adjustment for age-sex composition of the heart attack population (which is much older than the U.S. population) and for the fact that some reported heart attack deaths occurred in cases that had been readmitted, rather than truly new cases.

Heidenreich and McClellan contend that an even better indicator of the efficacy of treatment is the age-adjusted thirty-day fatality rate, which is influenced by treatment in the hospital and in the post-hospitalization period.[23] That rate has also fallen by 36 percent (table 1-2).

In summary, the age-adjusted population death rate from heart attacks declined by nearly 60 percent in the twenty-year period 1975–95 (see table 1-1). The age-sex adjusted thirty-day fatality rate for hospitalized cases fell by a little less than 40 percent (table 1-2). Although the two rates are not exactly comparable, it is clear that the improvement in heart attack mortality experience applies to both nonhospitalized and hospitalized cases, with a somewhat greater aggregate improvement in the cases when deaths occur outside hospitals.

For the phase they call "acute management," which encompasses the thirty-day interval of treatment after the onset of a heart attack, Cutler, McClellan, and Newhouse estimate that changes in the hospital treatments of heart attacks accounted for about 55 percent of the decline in acute-phase mortality. New or more widespread use of pharmaceutical treatments accounted for 50 percentage points of the total, by far the largest effects on heart attack mortality. The increased use of more invasive cardiac procedures (angioplasty and heart bypasses) accounted for a limited share of the reduction—only about 5 percent in their preferred estimate. Results from the medical literature cannot explain the other 45 percent of the reduction in the in-hospital death rate.[24]

Moreover, tables 1-1 and 1-2 tabulate only mortality. Heart disease affects the quality as well as the quantity of life, and the available evidence (see chapter 2, table 2-2) suggests improvements as well in the quality of life for heart disease sufferers.

23. Ibid.
24. Hunink and others (1997) reached similar conclusions for the decline in the death rate from coronary heart disease

Heart Attack Price Indexes

Although cardiovascular health has improved, expenditures for treating cardiovascular disease have soared. Nearly one-seventh of all medical spending is for cardiovascular disease, and that share has grown over time.[25] Medicare hospital spending per heart attack is nearly $15,000. With about 230,000 new heart attack cases annually, the Medicare program currently spends more than $3 billion on hospital care for heart attacks alone. Reductions in mortality have been gratifying; but was it worth the dramatic spending increases? Are we better off devoting resources to cardiovascular disease, or would we gain by reallocating resources elsewhere?

To answer these questions, Cutler, McClellan, and Newhouse first examine why Medicare spending on heart attacks has increased over time—from $11,000 per case in 1984 to $15,000 in 1991 (they adjusted both numbers for the overall rate of inflation). Using detailed claims records for the Medicare population, the researchers found that essentially all of the increased spending resulted from more intensive treatment of heart attacks.

For each type of heart attack treatment, the change in Medicare reimbursement was virtually identical to the overall inflation rate. Medicare spending rose more rapidly than the inflation rate because more patients received more intensive services, for which Medicare pays more, not because the rates for each of the services themselves rose faster than the general rate of inflation.

What were the health outcomes of increased treatment intensity? Were the increased expenditures worth it? To help answer those questions, Cutler, McClellan, and Newhouse computed price indexes for heart attack treatments that allowed for the value of the more intensive treatments that heart attack patients now receive. They compared the results with the CPI medical care component.

The authors appropriately emphasize a number of qualifications to the CPI comparisons they made. The CPI medical care component has a coverage that is broader than just heart attacks, and a price index for heart attacks is not necessarily representative of price indexes for all medical treatments. Additionally, because of data availability, Cutler, McClellan, and Newhouse computed price indexes from Medicare data for elderly heart attack victims and from heart attack cases in a large

---

25. Hodgson and Cohen (1998).

teaching hospital, whose name must be kept confidential. A price index for one hospital may not be representative of the entire country, and the cost experience of Medicare may not correspond very well to the medical care costs of non-Medicare, nonelderly patients. Nevertheless, when the authors mimicked CPI procedures on data from the major hospital, the two trend rates of change differed by only one-tenth (0.1) of a percentage point over the 1984–91 interval.

Although we should keep all those qualifications in mind, the Cutler, McClellan, and Newhouse results are provocative. In table 1-3, we have presented information from their table 2-10 in a slightly different form in order to bring out the implications of the research for BLS medical care price indexes.

As we noted earlier, the CPI is in concept a fixed-weight approximation to a cost-of-living index, and the CPI concept includes monetary, out-of-pocket expenditures only. The weights in the CPI formerly were held constant for a relatively long interval; the BLS used the average expenditure proportions in 1982–84 until early 1998. Before 1997, CPI medical components were constructed from a sample of standardized charges (a hospital room rate, for example). Cutler, McClellan, and New-house refer to that as a "service price index," although one might also call it a "price index for medical care inputs." The BLS now obtains prices for specified treatments for a particular disease. Cutler, McClellan, and New-house refer to that as a "treatment regimen price index."

The price index literature is dominated by concern that holding the weights unchanged might give an inflation measure that rises more than an index number that either adjusts the weighting structure more rapidly (usually referred to as a chain index) or one that uses a more complex index number formula that accommodates changes in consumers' market baskets of goods and services. One expects that the treatment regimen price index will rise less than the medical input price index if, for example, the number of hospital days required to treat a medical condition declines with improved medical methods.

The first part of table 1-3, which we base on Cutler, McClellan, and Newhouse's "major teaching hospital" price indexes, shows that both aspects of CPI implementation—pricing the inputs to medical care and holding the weights fixed—bias upward the price indexes for medical care. Holding the weights for medical inputs fixed at their 1984 proportions (which is roughly coincident with the CPI's former 1982–84 weighting period) creates an upward bias of 1.7 percentage points per year, compared with a chain price index that updates the weights annually. A

Table 1-3. *Sources of Bias in CPI Medical Care Price Index, Based on Estimates for Heart Attack Treatments*

Sources	Annual percentage points
On CPI's own concept (out-of-pocket, money expenditure only)	
Did not change weights in the CPI[a]	1.7
Priced inputs instead of treatment regimens[b]	0.3
Total bias, on CPI's own concept	2.0
On COL concept	
Did not allow for valuation of increased life expectancy[c]	1.1–1.5

Source: This volume, chapter 2, table 2-10.

a. 1984 weights index (line 3 in table 2-10) less annual chain weights index (line 4 in table 2-10).

b. Line 4 in table 2-10 less line 5.

c. Cost-of-living index line in table 2-10 less line 5 (range corresponds to alternative estimates of the COL index—see description in the text).

price index that is based on medical inputs creates an additional 0.3 percentage point of upward bias per year, compared with the treatment regimen price index, when both are computed on a chain basis.

Thus the constant-weight aspect of the old BLS method had an effect (1.7 points) that was much larger than the agency's former decision to price inputs rather than treatments (0.3 points). Economists will probably find that result surprising. As we noted earlier, one expects a substantial bias when the price index is formed from the hospital room rate or on the price for a doctor's office visit, because medical technology has reduced the length of hospital stays and because the doctor can now do more during that visit. The vision that pricing medical care inputs must bias the CPI upward has long been part of the health economist's tool bag. The Cutler, McClellan, and Newhouse research indicates that the vision is correct, but that it only accounts for a relatively small (0.3 percentage point) effect. Cutler, McClellan, and Newhouse's results suggest that the CPI could have been converted into a fairly effective cost-of-treatment price index simply—and cheaply—by frequently updating the weights attached to the medical inputs that it was pricing all along. Their finding that price index weights have a greater effect on medical price indexes than does technical change that reduces medical inputs per medical treatment is provocative and suggestive for future research on sources of measurement error in medical price indexes.

BLS materials emphasize that the CPI is an approximation to a cost-of-living index, albeit, as noted above, an approximation that is circum-

scribed in specific ways. One can also look at the price of medical treatments within the cost-of-living index framework. When we are dealing
with health, the way the cost-of-living index is defined matters.

For a cost-of-living index for goods—apples, oranges, carrots, and
cars—the consumer's monetary resources, monetary income or monetary
wealth, are what matters, mostly. It is true that nonmonetary costs also
exist for nonmedical consumption goods—for example, time costs for
shopping for apples and oranges, food preparation time for the carrots,
and driving time for use of the car. Economists have recognized, at least
since the work of Becker, that the omission of the consumer's time in
studies of consumption may neglect an important element that is necessary to analyze consumption behavior.[26] If the cost of time is essential to
analyze consumption behavior, it should also be accounted for in a cost-
of-living index. In the case of most consumption goods, neglecting time
and other nonmonetary costs has a long tradition, and staying within the
traditional market boundary that encloses money income and money
expenditures exclusively is deemed adequate for most purposes. For that
reason, the CPI concept has no room in it for the time required for any
consumption activity, or for improvements in any broader concept of
income or of consumption that the household does not receive in monetary terms.

In the case of health, and in some other services as well, it becomes
essential to go beyond the usual market or production boundary. One
seeks medical care for a heart attack to prolong life. Few individuals ask
explicitly: What is the value of the life for which I am purchasing medical
treatment? Yet, it is hard to understand the outcome of a medical treatment for heart attacks without considering the expected change in mortality that the patient expects from the treatment.

Additionally, if mortality change is a medical outcome measure that
needs to be brought into the price index calculation in some manner, it is
hard to see immediately how to do that without being willing to put a
value on the life so extended. Additional expenditures on apples and
oranges provide for more consumption of apples and oranges (even if
what is really wanted is, in some sense, nutrition). But no normal person
buys more medical care to consume more medical care; what one expects
to consume is more life or more health.

Accordingly, Cutler, McClellan, and Newhouse specify that a cost-of-
living index should measure "the increased spending on medical care

26. Becker (1960).

over time less the additional value of that care." To compute the value of improvements in heart attack care, they valued increased years of life expectancy for heart attack victims by an estimate of the value of an additional life-year, taken from economic estimates that were computed for other purposes. The researchers chose a value of $25,000 for an additional life-year, which is on the conservative side of current practice among economists.

Even with that low value, however, the researchers found that the benefits of increased survival (eight months at $25,000 per year, or about $12,000 in present value terms) are greater than the additional spending (about $4,000). Using a lower estimate of the change in life expectancy from improved medical treatments (four months) gave a lower estimate of the value, but one that was still well above the increment to medical costs. The lower estimate assumes that the entire Medicare population (heart attack victims and those who did not suffer a heart attack) enjoyed increased health from nonmedical sources, so that nonmedical factors caused part of the improvement in life expectancy for heart attack victims. The larger estimate assumes that improved medical care, for heart attacks and for other conditions, accounted for all the improvement in life expectancy.

As the "COL concept" row of table 1-3 shows, allowing for the value of increased life expectancy for heart attack victims lowered the cost-of-living index by 1.1–1.5 percentage points per year. The range corresponds to the two alternative assumptions, noted above, about sources of increased life expectancy in the Medicare population.

Cutler, McClellan, and Newhouse's cost-of-living index estimate has been controversial, mainly because many people are reluctant to put a value on additional years of life. Though the ethical reasons for that reluctance are well known, Triplett (chapter 7) contends that existing statistical methods for measuring medical price indexes implicitly contain the same assumption. The very nature of the economic problem—measuring the cost of medical treatments and the value of medical outcomes—forces such valuation.[27]

We noted earlier that third-party discounts have been an issue in measuring medical care prices. The discount effect is important to analyses that formerly used the CPI in the absence of a PPI index for the medical care industry. Estimates of discounts show the difference be-

27. For a similar view, see Gold and others (1996).

tween the CPI's out-of-pocket measure for consumers and what insurance companies and others were actually paying for medical services.[28]

Cutler, McClellan, and Newhouse used their hospital data to calculate the effect of discounts on the price index: 1.1 percentage points annually. As many medical economists suspected, discounts were rising substantially over the 1984–91 interval.

Whether discounts belong in the CPI is a somewhat complicated question that we need not discuss comprehensively here. The BLS includes consumer-purchased medical insurance in the CPI, and for that the information on discounts to third-party payers is relevant. Thus for the medical insurance part of the CPI, the total bias estimated by Cutler, McClellan, and Newhouse approximated 3.1 percentage points annually (2.0 percentage points on the out-of-pocket concept—see table 1-3—plus the 1.1 percentage points from industry discounts). But for the out-of-pocket medical expenditures portion of the CPI itself, discounts to third-party payers are not relevant.[29]

In summary, an important implication of the Cutler, McClellan, and Newhouse research is that the cost of restoring health for a person with a heart attack has risen less rapidly over time than has the general rate of inflation. The NBER research team estimated the decline in the cost of living, relative to the overall inflation rate, at about 1 percent annually. That is in sharp contrast to a conventional price index for heart attacks, which Cutler, McClellan, and Newhouse also computed from their data for the teaching hospital. This conventional price index increased more rapidly than the overall rate of inflation (about 3 percentage points more, annually). Accounting for the benefits (improved outcomes) of changing medical treatments thus has a fundamental impact on our view of the magnitude of price increases for medical care.

An Exploratory Analysis of Price Indexes for the Treatment of Acute Depression

What has happened to the cost of treating an episode of care for a common mental illness such as acute depression? Frank, Berndt, and Busch

28. Employer-provided medical insurance has always been outside the scope of the CPI definition of consumption.

29. One could also argue that the full cost-of-living index, to which the CPI is an approximation, ought to include in its consumption measure the medical services purchased by employer-provided medical insurance. This debate takes us too far into the details of price index construction.

(chapter 3) find that the cost of treating acute depression to guideline standards of care has fallen during the 1990s. The recent increase in mental health expenditures therefore reflects very substantial growth in the quantity of treatments for depression and not in the price of those treatments.

Treatments for major depression have advanced rapidly over the past twenty years. Innovative techniques in psychotherapy include interpersonal therapy, behavior therapy, family therapy, and cognitive behavior therapy. Each of those treatments has been shown to reduce depressive symptoms for less severe forms of major depression at comparable efficacy and with similar outcomes. Innovative advances in antidepressant pharmaceuticals have been dramatic as well, especially since the introduction of the selective serotonin reuptake inhibitors (SSRIs) in 1988. The SSRIs are associated with significantly fewer side effects and are easier to take than the older generation of tricyclic antidepressants (TCAs). In treating major depression, doctors frequently combine psychotherapeutic interventions with antidepressant medications.

Using guidelines published by the Agency for Health Care Policy Research and the American Psychiatric Association, Frank, Berndt, and Busch identified nine major sets of "treatment bundles" for acute depression that employ various mixes of psychotherapy, antidepressant drugs, and medical management. They identified those bundles by using criteria based on data from clinical trials. Thus the episodes of care the authors considered corresponded directly to treatments tested in the clinical trial literature. The researchers constructed medical price indexes based on the cost of treating an entire episode of acute depression in a manner that met published treatment guidelines.

A notable initial finding was that only 15–25 percent of episodes of depression treatment met guideline standards. The authors compute prices only for those treatment episodes meeting guideline standards. They noted that in subsequent research they will relax the "pure" definition of an episode of care, thereby pricing an episode of care that more realistically captures actual treatments.[30]

The researchers' review of the clinical trial and medical literature revealed the following conclusions regarding expected outcomes from those various treatment bundles:

—Compared with no treatment, psychotherapies of all kinds result in superior outcomes.

30. Subsequent research, not reported here, determined that the price indexes were in fact sensitive to whether or not the patient received the full guideline level of care.

—Psychotherapies alone, TCAs with medical management, TCAs alone, and SSRIs alone appear to produce comparable outcomes for less severe forms of major depression in terms of short-term symptom reduction.

—For more severe forms of major depression, TCAs alone, SSRIs alone, and combinations of drugs and psychotherapy have comparable levels of efficacy.

—Compared with TCAs, SSRI use is associated with a higher rate of achieving recommended lengths of treatment.

To develop prices for treatment bundles, Frank, Berndt, and Busch relied on outpatient and pharmaceutical claims data from the Medicaid Statistical Reporting and Analysis System, which were drawn from four large self-insured employers covering about a half-million people annually from 1991 through 1995. Those claims data are associated with alternative treatment bundles meeting published guideline standards of care. The researchers found that prices received by providers differed markedly across treatment bundles. Even for therapeutically similar treatment bundles, for example, prices in 1993 ranged from $254 for short-term SSRI treatment alone to $924 for short-term psychotherapy alone.

Alternative Price Indexes for the Treatment of Acute Depression

Prices of alternative treatment bundles for each year over the 1991–95 time period provided the basis for constructing alternative price indexes for treating depression. Price measures for the treatment of acute major depression were computed in several different ways. One price measure, analogous to the PPI, is based on the total revenues received by the provider—the sum of the insurers' payments plus those of the patient. Another, analogous to the CPI, is based only on the direct payments made by the patient for treatment—copayments plus deductibles.

Frank, Berndt, and Busch computed price indexes under a variety of assumptions. In one case, they computed the price index based on the assumption that the treatment bundles could not be substituted for one another. That index conforms to the Laspeyres formula used by the BLS. In another, they considered various treatment bundles to be perfectly substitutable. Their final price index used an index number formula (the Tornqvist) endorsed by the CPI Commission.[31] That index incorporates the changing value shares of the various bundles over time and made no

---

31. Boskin and others (1996).

a priori assumption concerning the substitutability of the various treatment bundles, so the index represents a "compromise" of the two extreme assumptions about substitutability.

No matter how they constructed the index, Frank, Berndt, and Busch
found that the price of treating acute major depression fell by close to 30
percent over the 1991–95 time period (price declines of roughly 7 percent
per year). In the PPI-like index, the 1991–95 price decline ranged from
22 to 30 percent.

Price declines of this magnitude imply that the recent increases in
mental health care expenditures involve a substantial growth in the quantity of treatments and not in their prices. Price declines reflect the price
concessions won by the rapidly growing managed-care sector, as well as
the changing mix of treatment bundles—increasing the prescription pharmaceutical component and SSRI use and reducing the intensity of psychotherapy, which is by far the most expensive form of treatment.

Although no exact match exists among published PPI and CPI price
indexes, the most closely related components of those indexes all rose
over the period. For example, the inpatient treatment PPI rose about 10
percent and the medical care services CPI more than 25 percent over the
same interval. The authors conclude: "Our results [suggest] that the
[medical] CPI and PPIs may be particularly prone to distortion . . . where
managed care has potentially large impacts on both input prices and the
composition of treatment and there has been important technical change
in treatment methods."

An Exploratory Study of Price Indexes for Cephalosporins

Sara Ellison and Judith Hellerstein (chapter 4) have produced price
indexes for the cephalosporin class of antibiotics—a large and important
subclass of antibiotics indicated for a wide range of infections—that are
used in different clinical settings. They computed price indexes for
branded and generic cephalosporins, distinguished separately cephalosporins sold across different channels of distribution, and compared those
new price indexes with the cephalosporins component of the PPI. The
researchers report that their new price indexes rose less rapidly than the
PPI indexes. Measured by the new price indexes, the average annual
increase in cephalosporin prices was modest—only .76 percent, compared
with a 4.54 percent average annual increase in the cephalosporins PPI.

The Ellison-Hellerstein study adds to the existing body of NBER
research suggesting that a significant upward bias existed in the prescrip-

tion drug PPI under the old BLS methodology. As we noted earlier, however, the BLS has recently made significant changes in both the PPI and CPI programs to correct for bias caused by not linking generics and by oversampling older products and undersampling newer prescription drugs.[32] An important topic for future research will be the extent to which the new procedures employed by the BLS have eliminated the upward bias existing under the old methodology.

Although the slow growth in those cephalosporins price indexes indicates that antibiotics have remained inexpensive, Ellison and Hellerstein note that those price data mask one other very significant cost-saving feature of antibiotics. In the past, certain bacterial infections led to routine hospitalizations for some segments of the population (for example, very young children). To the extent that antibiotics now keep people out of the hospital when they contract a bacterial infection, the price of treating bacterial infections has become much lower, both because the direct cost is lower and because the indirect cost—the emotional and developmental cost of hospitalizing young children—is reduced. That extra cost saving from substituting outpatient treatment with antibiotics for hospital care is not reflected in the pharmaceutical price indexes computed by the authors. In a sense, pharmaceuticals are inputs to the production of medical care. Although it is extraordinarily important to get the inputs measured correctly, in the end we want to know the costs of what the pharmaceuticals do to health conditions and the contribution they make to improving health and to reducing the cost of health care.

The Economics of Antibiotics and Drug Patents and Prices

Two studies, in addition to addressing price measurement, considered the economic incentives for developing new pharmaceuticals and for generating adequate information about medical outcomes for new and for existing pharmaceuticals.

Ellison and Hellerstein (chapter 4) developed an economic model of the incentives for research on new antibiotics. Seventy years ago, bacterial infections such as pneumonia, tuberculosis, and typhoid fever were leading causes of death worldwide. Although McKeown and his collaborators demonstrated that in industrialized countries the decline in the death rates from those diseases began long before the development of

32. Kelly (1997).

effective antibacterial pharmaceuticals,[33] treatment with readily available and inexpensive antibiotics has now essentially eradicated typhoid fever in the developed world and reduced most cases of pneumonia and tuberculosis to readily curable conditions. Ellison and Hellerstein point out that when an antibiotic is used successfully to combat an infectious disease, the benefit accrues not only to the person who takes the antibiotic but to other persons who, if the antibiotic were not used, might have contracted the contagious disease. Thus individuals who do not have the disease have an interest in promoting more use of antibiotics to reduce their probabilities of contracting it. However, their interests are not factored into the decision to take the antibiotic. In the language of economics, this is an externality that results in too small a value being placed on the antibiotic and too little of it being used.

On the other hand, more use of an existing antibiotic increases the probability of bacterial resistance to it, which makes the drug less effective in the future. In that case, Ellison and Hellerstein contend that private decisionmakers will fail to make sufficient use of a diversity of antibiotics, which also reduces the demand for *new* antibiotics. Their study does not estimate the magnitudes of those two effects.

Thomas Croghan, Patricia Danzon, and Henry Grabowski (comments to chapter 4) find Ellison and Hellerstein's model somewhat rudimentary, at its current stage, to be fully convincing. Each had somewhat different reasons. Croghan points out that the model was not realistic for medical reasons. Danzon notes that the model did not consider adequately at its current stage the distinction between broad-spectrum antibiotics and narrower-spectrum ones; incentives to produce drugs with excessively broad spectrums might be too great, so the model might have been misleading. Grabowski adds that the Ellison-Hellerstein model did not consider alternatives, such as vaccines to prevent disease. Incentives to develop preventive drugs (vaccines) may be too low for a variety of reasons he listed, including federal government action, and one cannot determine whether the incentives to produce antibiotics are nonoptimal without considering as well alternative medical courses of action against infectious diseases.

Thus Crogan, Danzon, and Grabowski contend that the Ellison-Hellerstein model's results were very sensitive to special assumptions that the authors made. Though those criticisms were telling, formal economic models are always dependent on their assumptions, and the early stage

33. McKeown (1976).

of modeling on most economic problems frequently leaves substantial room for subsequent improvement. The Ellison-Hellerstein model was no different from others in that respect, and it is best viewed as an interesting start on a difficult economic problem.

Joel Hay and Winnie Yu (chapter 5) emphasize that a large proportion of our information about the effectiveness of pharmaceuticals is based on clinical trials sponsored by manufacturers of patented pharmaceuticals. That, they argue, creates a bias in incentives, because some kinds of pharmaceutical knowledge can be patented, whereas for others a patent cannot be obtained.

For example, if a new use is discovered for an old drug (an example might be the discovery that aspirin was an effective drug for treating heart attacks), one cannot obtain a patent for that discovery because the drug itself has long since passed the limits on patent protection. Thus, Hay and Yu contend, pharmaceutical firms have no incentive to develop new information about the usefulness of "old" drugs, which implies that private research resources are biased toward the development of new (and patentable) drugs, even when society might be better off putting resources into the exploration of the properties of known chemical compounds. Hay and Yu present quite a number of anecdotes to make their point. They proposed an expansion of use patents to change the present incentive structure.

While conceding the bias to private research incentives that Hay and Yu point out, Crogan, Danzon, and Grabowski (comments to chapter 5) raise an impressive number of objections to the desirability and feasibility of the Hay-Yu use-patents proposal. For example, both Croghan and Grabowski point out that use patents already exist but that enforcing a patent on the use of a drug, rather than on the right to manufacture it, requires producers to sue infringing physicians, HMOs, and patients. Grabowski wryly notes "the disinclination on the part of firms to sue their customers." Crogan, Danzon, and Grabowski also cite some undesirable incentive effects that the Hay-Yu use-patent proposal would create.

Additionally, defects in private-sector incentives to produce new knowledge on older drugs might be remedied by publicly funded research rather than by trying to improve private-sector incentives to carry out research that is not profitable. Hay and Yu, however, dismissed the latter possibility because, they contend, the National Institutes of Health are "limited by competing demands for medical research initiatives, the micro- and macropolitics of bioscientific research and development resource allocation decisions across diseases and therapies, the dogma of prevailing scientific paradigms, the prejudices and political correctness of academic experts, and the red tape of government bureaucracy."

The use-patent proposal is not, in itself, directly relevant to the topic of measuring the prices of medical treatments.

Cost, Effects, Outcomes, and Utility and Integrating Price Index and Cost-Effectiveness Research

Two studies dealt with the broad view: How can one combine research on measuring medical care into an overall economic picture of medical inflation, the quantity and quality of medical treatments, and the consumption of medical care?

Pauly (chapter 6) proposes an alternative to the approach taken in the empirical studies in this volume. Rather than measure the price of medical treatments with appropriate quality adjustments, he proposed to measure the change in willingness to pay for insured medical services: "My suggestion is that the *object* of valuation be defined as the difference between the willingness to pay premiums for a managed care plan covering of the technology available in the preceding period and the willingness to pay for the same plan covering the technology available in the current period."

As Pauly notes, pricing medical care by pricing insurance plans was proposed at least thirty years ago.[34] What is new, Pauly contends, is the development of willingness-to-pay techniques in economics. Now, one could ask respondents to put a valuation on an insurance policy that covered some new technique, or a bundle of new techniques, compared with an insurance policy that did not cover those techniques.

One advantage of pricing insurance policies is that such an approach captures behavior toward risk in a way that is perhaps neglected in studies that only address the cost of treating a disease. If one has a disease, and if there is no insurance, the cost of treating the disease matters. If one does not have the disease, then insuring against the risk of a costly medical bill if the disease is contracted is important.

Pauly points out that in the United States insurance covers some 80 percent of medical expenses. For the insured population, the cost of treating a disease is not quite what matters, in the sense of computing, say, a cost-of-living index for medical care. Instead, Pauly contends, a cost-of-living index should include the cost of medical insurance.

34. Reder (1969).

Pauly buttresses his case for pricing insurance by discussing many of the problems that arise in constructing quality-adjusted life-years (QALY), which is an essential component of the alternative approach proposed by Triplett (chapter 7). He concludes, "The advantage of this method [QALY] then is not its credibility."

There is little question that Pauly's list of problems with measuring QALY consists of legitimate concerns. Indeed, one can find similar discussions in the QALY literature itself. For example, the report of Gold and others, in which QALY was proposed as the standard medical outcome measure for cost-effectiveness studies, contains an extensive discussion of the primitive stage of development of the QALY measure and the problems that have yet to be resolved.[35]

In addition, Pauly makes a new point about the use of QALY in price indexes. For most cost-effectiveness studies—the purpose for which QALYs are usually computed—finding a precise value for QALY is not required. All that is necessary, in most cases, is to determine whether cost per QALY is below some threshold number or to compare cost per QALY for two or more alternative treatments. For those purposes, a precise measure of QALY is not necessary because there are few "close calls" for which real precision matters.

In the case of price indexes, however, using QALY as a measure of medical outcome to make an adjustment for changes in medical technology requires, in principle, a precise measure. Even when more QALY estimates become available, they may not be measured precisely enough to meet the needs of economic statistics.

Pauly concludes that a mix of pricing insurance and use of QALY may be appropriate: "For analysis of expenditure changes for populations heavily subsidized by public programs—Medicaid and the part of Medicare spending that goes to low-income elderly—it may be best to use the monetized QALYs approach, precisely because the monetization, as well as the entire program, is really an object of collective choice. There is little point, say, in adjusting Medicaid spending for the value Medicaid beneficiaries place on improved quality, even if we knew it."

Triplett's study (chapter 7) focuses on an augmented national health account that would better accommodate research on medical prices and medical outcomes. He proposes integrating the present national health accounts constructed by HCFA with the "cost of disease" accounts origi-

35. Gold and others (1996).

nally constructed by Rice, and recently implemented in expanded form by Hodgson and Cohen.[36] Cost-of-disease accounts already disaggregate total expenditures on medical care by disease classifications (International Classification of Diseases, 9th revision, or ICD-9). For example, ICD-9, chapter 7, covers circulatory diseases, including heart attacks—the focus of the Cutler, McClellan, and Newhouse study. Triplett remarks that organizing health accounts by disease classifications (rather than, as now, by source and recipient of funds) is analogous to the "product" side of conventional national accounts, because funds are spent on diseases.

Estimating real output of medical care in Triplett's augmented national health account system could proceed by using the new PPI medical care indexes that are already arranged by Diagnostic Related Groups (DRGs). DRGs are consistent, for the most part, with ICD-9 classifications. Triplett also contends that it would be natural and straightforward to build into the deflation process new research on price indexes by disease, as it became available. For example, the price indexes for heart attacks and for mental depression contained in this volume, and the Shapiro and Wilcox study of cataract surgery, could be substituted for PPI indexes, or they could be used to supplement them.[37] New research could be integrated piece by piece as new studies become available.

Additionally, the burgeoning growth of cost-effectiveness studies provides information about medical outcomes that could be also used in a systematic way if the national health accounts were organized by ICD-9 classifications rather than, as now, by sources of funding and recipients of funds. Triplett notes that the approach outlined in his study could be implemented in countries where no private markets for medical care or for medical insurance exist, which is a great advantage for future international comparisons of medical costs and real consumption of medical care.

To execute such an expanded health account system, one needs to understand how price indexes for medical care and cost-effectiveness studies fit together. Triplett's study explains the relationships between those two bodies of research. This technical demonstration matters for practical purposes when and if an accounting for health care is established that can make use of both new price index studies and new cost-effectiveness studies as they become available.

---

36. See Levit and others (1996) on the national health accounts constructed by HCFA; Rice (1966) and Hodgson and Cohen (1998) on cost of disease accounts.
37. Shapiro and Wilcox (1996).

Neither Pauly nor Triplett proposes one approach to the exclusion of the other. Indeed, the real problem is that both approaches have difficulties and too little information is available for implementing either approach.

On the Pauly insurance proposal, Weisbrod (chapter 8) notes that "health insurance contracts are not available now with coverage limited to services that were available at some prior time."

With respect to Triplett's use of information from cost-effectiveness analysis, Hay and Yu (chapter 5) maintain that not only is the information currently available insufficient, but also too few incentives exist to produce more of it. Pauly, as well as Manning (chapter 8) and Meltzer (chapter 8), points out inherent problems with QALY and some of the difficulties in using QALY to construct better price indexes.

Probably the best way to look at this debate is to say that there are two glasses of water, both of which are nearly empty. If either one were close to full (with empirical studies), it could be used effectively to improve measures of medical care. Pauly finds conceptual reasons for preferring that the glass marked "measuring insurance policies" be the one into which the refreshing water of empirical research be poured. Triplett points out that the springs of new research are now filling the other glass. Even if there is now the sediment that others claim to see in the glass (because of problems with QALY and so forth), he expects the filters to be improved as the glass is filled (methods will be improved as more research is done). He therefore opts to build a conceptual framework that will make use of the studies that are accumulating rather than to wait for researchers to implement the price-of-insurance approach.

Conclusion

An encouraging number of new developments in measuring medical care have occurred very recently. Most of them are not yet well known. Together, they are changing our perceptions of medical care inflation and of the quantity of medical care services provided by U.S. expenditure on medical care.

Statistical agencies have greatly improved government price indexes for medical care—for medical care providers, such as hospitals and physicians, and also for pharmaceuticals. Some of these PPI and CPI improvements are the direct result of previous research into new methods for medical care price index measurement, particularly by a group of NBER researchers.

The papers in this volume also present promising new developments in measuring medical care. New methodologies and new empirical estimates for selected medical care disease categories suggest that improvements in medical care are greater than the usual statistics suggest and that medical care price inflation is lower. The papers and discussion also offer insights into future directions for research.

It is also true that the contributions in this volume suggest how much is yet to be done. Only a small number of medical procedures have been studied intensively. One cannot infer that price indexes for heart attacks, depression, and antibiotics are representative of what researchers will find when studies are completed for other medical procedures. Even though much that is promising has occurred very recently, it is still too soon to see how the full economic picture of medical care will look when more of the pieces have been studied.

There is good news, though: Progress is being made. That is the story of this volume.

References

Becker, Gary S. 1965. "A Theory of the Allocation of Time." *Economic Journal* 75 (September): 493–517.

Berndt, Ernst R., Zvi Griliches, and Joshua G. Rosett. 1993. "Auditing the Producer Price Index: Micro Evidence from Prescription Pharmaceutical Preparations." *Journal of Business and Economic Statistics* 11(3) (July): 251–64.

Boskin, Michael J., and others. December 4, 1996. "Toward a More Accurate Measure of the Cost of Living: Final Report to the Senate Finance Committee from the Advisory Commission to Study the Consumer Price Index."

Gold, Marthe R., and others. 1996. *Cost-Effectiveness in Health and Medicine*. New York: Oxford University Press.

Griliches, Zvi, and Iain Cockburn. 1994. "Generics and New Goods in Pharmaceutical Price Indexes." *American Economic Review* 84(5) (December): 1213–32.

Heidenreich, Paul, and Mark McClellan. 1998. "Trends in Heart Attack Treatment and Outcomes, 1975–1995: A Literature Review and Synthesis," in a volume edited by Ernst R. Berndt and David Cutler emanating from the Conference on Research in Income and Wealth, June 1998 (forthcoming).

Hodgson, Thomas A., and Alan J. Cohen. 1998. "Medical Care Expenditures for Major Diseases." Manuscript. National Center for Health Statistics, Hyattsville, Md.

Hunink, Maria G. M., and others. 1997. "The Recent Decline in Mortality from Coronary Heart Disease, 1980–1990: The Effect of Secular Trends in Risk Factors and Treatment." *Journal of the American Medical Association* 277(7): 535–42.

Kanoza, Douglas. 1996. "Supplemental Sampling in the PPI Pharmaceuticals Index." *Producer Price Indexes Detailed Price Report* (January): 8–10.

Kelly, Gregory G. 1997. "Improving the PPI Samples for Prescription Pharmaceuticals." *Monthly Labor Review* 120(10) (October): 10–17.

Levit, Katherine R., and others. 1996. "National Health Expenditures, 1995." *Health Care Financing Review* 18(1): 175–214.

McKeown, Thomas. 1976. *The Role of Medicine: Dream, Mirage, or Nemesis?* London: Nuffield Provincial Hospitals Trust.

Newhouse, Joseph P. 1989. "Measuring Medical Prices and Understanding Their Effects—The Baxter Prize Address." *Journal of Health Administration Education* 7(1): 19–26.

Reder, M. W. 1969. "Some Problems in the Measurement of Productivity in the Medical Care Industry." In *Production and Productivity in the Service Industries*, edited by Victor R. Fuchs. National Bureau of Economic Research Studies in Income and Wealth, vol. 34, pp. 95–131. Columbia University Press.

Rice, Dorothy P. 1966. *Estimating the Cost of Illness.* Government Printing Office.

Ristow, William. 1996. IMS presentation to the BLS. Mimeo. IMS America, Plymouth Meeting, Pa. (July).

Shapiro, Matthew P., and David W. Wilcox. 1996. "Mismeasurement in the Consumer Price Index: An Evaluation." *NBER Macroeconomics Annual* 11: 93–142.

U.S. Department of Commerce, Bureau of Economic Analysis. 1985. *Introduction to National Economic Accounting.* Methodology Paper series MP-1. Government Printing Office.

———. 1990. "Improving the Quality of Economic Statistics." *Survey of Current Business* 70(2) (February): 2.

U.S. Department of Health and Human Services. 1989. *The International Classification of Diseases, 9th Revision, Clinical Modification: ICD-9-CM.* 3d ed. Vols. 1–3. U.S. Department of Health and Human Services, Public Health Service, Health Care Financing Administration.

U.S. Department of Health and Human Services, National Center for Health Statistics. 1995. *Vital and Health Statistics: National Hospital Discharge Survey: Annual Summary, 1993,* 13(121) (August): 62.

———. 1997. *Monthly Vital Statistics Report* 45(11) (supplement 2) (June 12).

U.S. Department of Labor, Bureau of Labor Statistics. Not dated. *Improvements to CPI Procedures: Prescription Drugs.*

2

The Costs and Benefits of Intensive Treatment for Cardiovascular Disease

David Cutler, Mark McClellan, and Joseph Newhouse

CARDIOVASCULAR DISEASE is among the most important health problems in the United States. Table 2-1 shows the leading causes of death in the United States in 1994. Heading the list is cardiovascular disease—diseases of the heart and cerebrovascular disease. The annual mortality rate from cardiovascular disease is a little over 0.3 percent. Second in importance—but only 60 percent as large—is cancer. Chronic obstructive pulmonary disease is a distant third. The high mortality from cardiovascular disease is indicative of its enormous economic burden. Recent estimates have put the burden of cardiovascular disease in the United States at $110 billion annually, and cardiovascular disease is projected to become the leading cause of death in the world over the next several decades. Indeed, the prominence of cardiovascular disease in mortality has been true for some time: it has been the leading cause of death in the United States since the turn of the century.

What is striking about mortality from cardiovascular disease, however, is not just its magnitude but how rapidly it has declined over time. Figure 2-1 shows age-adjusted cardiovascular disease mortality from 1950 to 1994. Cardiovascular disease mortality fell by 60 percent between 1950 and 1990.[1] The decline is pronounced and continues to this day.

We are grateful to Ernie Berndt and Zvi Griliches for helpful comments and to the Bureau of Economic Analysis, the Bureau of Labor Statistics, Eli Lilly, and the National Institutes on Aging for research support.

1. The values in figure 2-1 are adjusted to the age distribution of the population in 1950, and thus do not match the data in table 2-1, which uses the 1990 population.

Table 2-1. *Leading Causes of Death in the United States, 1995*

Deaths per 100,000 people

Cause	Death rate
Cardiovascular disease	341.4
Diseases of heart	281.2
Cerebrovascular disease	60.2
Malignant neoplasms	204.7
Chronic obstructive pulmonary disease	39.9
Accidents and adverse effects	34.1
Pneumonia and influenza	31.8
Diabetes mellitus	22.5
HIV	16.2
Suicide	11.8
Chronic liver disease and cirrhosis	9.5
Total	880.0

Source: National Center for Health Statistics (1997).

Not only is mortality falling, but the health of cardiovascular disease survivors is improving as well. Table 2-2 shows changes in functional status for people diagnosed with ischemic heart disease.[2] Over the past two decades, the share of people whose usual activity was limited by ischemic heart disease fell rapidly, and the share with no limitations rose. The percentage of people reporting overall poor health also fell.

In this chapter, we focus on this dramatic improvement in cardiovascular health and its implications for understanding the medical sector. Knowing just that cardiovascular health has improved is not enough; understanding the importance of this trend requires asking several other questions as well: Why has cardiovascular health improved? Has the money spent on cardiovascular disease care been "worth it"? How are changes in the medical sector affecting this benefit-cost calculation?

We analyze in particular the costs and benefits of care for heart attacks—a major and particularly severe form of cardiovascular disease. We direct our attention to heart attacks for several reasons. First, heart attacks are a common form of cardiovascular disease and among its most serious consequences; thus mortality will be a good measure of outcomes. Heart attacks are also expensive. Medicare spends over $14,000 per patient on hospital bills alone in the year after a heart attack, plus additional amounts for physicians and outpatient care. Further, these

2. These numbers are taken from various Health Interview Surveys. See Cutler and Richardson (1997) for more discussion as well as age adjustments.

Figure 2-1. *Cardiovascular Disease Mortality, 1950–94*

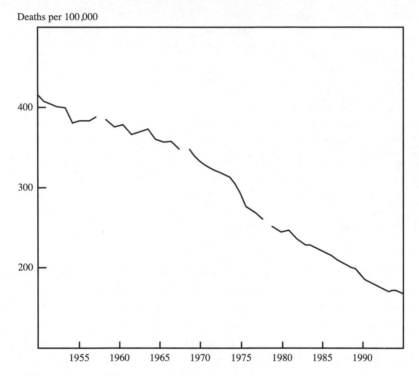

Deaths per 100,000

Source: Authors' calculations based on data from the National Center for
Health Statistics.

costs have been increasing at a rate of 4 percent per year in real (relative
to the GDP deflator) per capita terms. By analyzing the value of heart
attack treatment, we can learn a great deal about the costs and benefits of medical care in a situation of rapidly rising spending. Finally,
data to analyze heart attack treatments are easier to obtain than are
data for other cardiovascular conditions or other medical conditions
more generally.

Our analysis addresses four specific questions. The questions, and the
answers that we give, are:

1. What factors have led to reduced mortality for heart attack sufferers over time?

To address this question, we have undertaken a comprehensive literature review of publications in the last fifteen years addressing trends in
AMI (acute myocardial infarction, or heart attack) patient characteris-

Table 2-2. *Changes in Functional Status for People Reporting Having Been Diagnosed with Ischemic Heart Disease*

Percent

Measure	1972	1981	1982	1991
Functional limitations resulting from IHD[a]				
Cannot perform usual activity	16.7	15.5	15.0	8.6
Can perform usual activity but limited in amount and kind	29.0	21.3	12.3	6.3
Can perform usual activity but limited in outside activities	6.6	5.2	8.4	7.6
Not limited or ischemic heart disease not primary cause	47.8	58.0	64.3	77.5
Self-reported health status[b]				
Excellent	...	...	4.5	5.2
Very good	...	...	12.2	12.1
Good	...	...	26.5	27.1
Fair	...	...	28.2	29.8
Poor	...	...	28.0	24.9

Source: Data are from the Health Interview Surveys.

a. After 1981 the wording changed to: unable to perform major activity; limited in kind/amount of major activity; limited in other activities; and not limited.

b. Self-reported health status was not asked prior to 1982.

tics, treatments, outcomes, and costs of care between 1975 and 1995. We find that changes in acute treatments such as use of aspirin, beta blockers, thrombolytic drugs, and (to a limited extent) invasive procedures account for a substantial part of the improvement in mortality. Trends in "secondary prevention" have also probably contributed to improved health, although population data on trends in secondary prevention are sketchy and distinguishing these effects from long-term consequences of changes in acute treatment is difficult. Changes in individual risk factors related to behavior rather than medical technology have played only a limited role. These findings are confirmed by our analysis of medical claims and outcomes measures for Medicare beneficiaries suffering a heart attack.

2. What accounts for the rapid increase in the cost of heart attack care over time?

Using data on everyone in the Medicare population with a heart attack between 1984 and 1991, as well as heart attack records from a major teaching hospital between 1983 and 1995, we find that increasing costs of heart attack care are due almost entirely to increasing intensity of medical treatments. Reimbursement for a given type of therapy has been essentially unchanged.

3. How do the costs of increasing technology in heart attack care compare to the benefits of that care?

We estimate that between 1984 and 1991, life expectancy after a heart attack rose by eight months. Assuming rather conservative values for the benefit of additional life-years, the dollar value of this additional life is greater than the increased costs of medical care. This finding implies that the cost-of-living index for heart attack episodes fell, most likely by 1 percent or more annually.

4. How will changes in the medical care environment, particularly the growth of managed care, affect the nature of heart attack treatment?

When we compare heart attack patients treated in managed care and fee-for-service settings, we find that managed care plans in Massachusetts spend substantially less on heart attack care than fee-for-service plans. The cost difference is almost entirely a result of differences in the prices paid for equivalent care rather than differences in the quantity of care received.

The Nature of Cardiovascular Disease

The path of cardiovascular disease is depicted in figure 2-2. People initially engage in actions or have other diseases that place them at risk of a major cardiovascular illness. The most important risk factors are high blood pressure, high levels of cholesterol, smoking, obesity, and diabetes.[3]

Some people with elevated risk for cardiovascular illness (and some whose risk is not elevated) will suffer a serious cardiovascular event. These events include acute myocardial infarction, atherosclerosis, and cerebrovascular disease (stroke). A heart attack is a death of the heart muscle caused by blockage of the coronary arteries supplying blood to the heart. Longer-term consequences of these illnesses include congestive heart failure (chronic weakening of the heart muscle). The process of preventing individuals with or without known risk factors from developing serious illness is termed primary prevention.

For an individual who suffers a major cardiovascular illness, there is a period of acute disease management, which generally lasts about ninety days, although many critical treatments are delivered in the first few hours after the heart attack begins, and some therapies may be provided for up to several years after the event. Figure 2-3 shows the potential acute-phase treatments for patients with a heart attack. One treatment

---

3. Braunwald (1997); Hunink and others (1997).

Figure 2-2. *Cardiovascular Disease Progression*

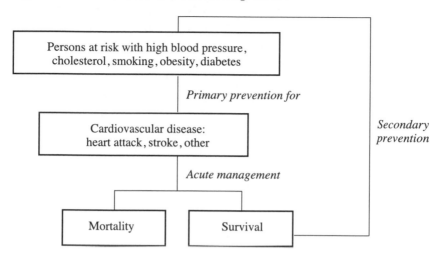

method involves medical management of the heart attack. In the acute period, medical management includes cardiopulmonary resuscitation, drug therapies such as aspirin administration to prevent clot expansion and thrombolysis to dissolve the clot, monitoring technologies, and other nonsurgical intensive interventions for complications such as heart failure and irregular heart rhythms. Later it may include drug therapy and counseling to promote a healthy lifestyle and reduce the risk of future heart attacks.

Figure 2-3. *Treatment of Patients with a Heart Attack*

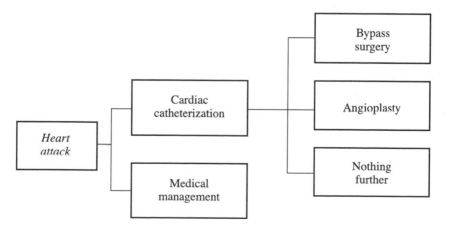

Invasive treatments for heart disease begin with cardiac catheterization, a diagnostic radiologic study of blood flow to the heart muscle.[4] If a catheterization detects significant blockage, a range of revascularization procedures may be applied. Two major types of revascularization procedures have become widely used: bypass surgery, a major open-heart operation that involves bypassing blocked blood vessels by splicing a vein or artery around the blockage, and angioplasty, a percutaneous, or less-invasive, procedure that seeks to restore blood flow by inflating a balloon amid the blockage.

If the individual survives the acute phase, a period of secondary prevention and complication management follows, designed to prevent the recurrence of an acute episode as well as to minimize any functional consequences of heart damage from the attack. The factors involved in secondary prevention are the same as those in primary prevention—managing blood pressure and cholesterol and encouraging weight reduction and exercise. Secondary prevention is particularly important, however, because individuals who have had a heart attack are at considerably higher risk of additional damage from the progression of heart disease. In addition, if the heart is weakened after the initial attack, medical treatments to support heart failure may be beneficial.

Sources of Health Improvement

Improvements in cardiovascular mortality and morbidity have resulted from a combination of primary prevention, acute disease management, and secondary prevention and complication management. All of these factors involve both medical and nonmedical components. The important question is how to parcel out these different effects and, in particular, how to gauge the importance of medical and nonmedical interventions in improved cardiovascular health.

The introduction of many primary and secondary therapies is at least coincident with the reduction in cardiovascular disease mortality. Table 2-3 shows key dates in the introduction of many pharmaceuticals used in cardiovascular care. Although cardioprotective effects of several drugs have been known for some time, most of the major drug treatments used

4. We define "invasive" treatments as catheterization and revascularization procedures. Many other "medical" treatments of AMI are also invasive, strictly speaking, but considerably less so than catheterization and revascularization.

Table 2-3. *Dates of Introduction of Important Pharmaceuticals for Cardiovascular Care*

Drug class	Year of innovation[a]
Antihypertensives	1959
Beta blockers	1962
Calcium-channel blockers	1971
ACE inhibitors	1979

Source: Food and Drug Administration calculations.

a. The year of innovation refers to the first drug in the class. Other advances were made in later years.

for ischemic heart disease have been developed since the 1950s.[5] The first oral diuretics (for blood pressure reduction) were introduced in 1959. Beta blockers (to reduce the heart's workload) were first developed in 1962, calcium-channel blockers (which also reduce heart workload through effects on cardiac contractions) were initially developed in 1971, and ACE inhibitors (angiotension converting enzyme inhibitors, which reduce the "afterload" facing the heart) were initially developed in 1979. Over the years, many modified versions of all of these compounds have been developed, with intended goals of improving effectiveness and reducing side effects of the treatments.

Innovation in acute care management has also been rapid. Table 2-4 shows the major technologies used in the treatment of major cardiovascular events (including AMI and heart failure) and when they were introduced. Cardiac catheterization was first performed in 1959, and open-heart surgery was initially developed in 1968. The 1970s saw the advent of cardiac intensive care units (ICUs), and thrombolytic drugs, first developed in the 1970s, began to be more widely applied in the 1980s. Use of angioplasty, first developed in 1978, spread in the 1980s and 1990s. In addition to these technologies, many other "technologies" are relevant to acute treatment, including the provision of basic and advanced cardiac life support, the expertise of emergency medical technicians (EMTs), paramedics, and other emergency response personnel, and the specialization of nursing care for cardiac cases.

There is substantial debate about the importance of different factors in explaining reductions in cardiovascular disease mortality. Most likely all of them have been important, and their significance is likely to have

5. Nitroglycerin was first used to treat angina pectoris in 1879, and digitalis use for heart failure also dates back to the nineteenth century.

Table 2-4. *Dates of Introduction of Important Advances for Acute Treatment of Cardiovascular Disease*

Treatment	Year of innovation[a]
Catheterization	1959
Coronary bypass	1968
Cardiac ICUs	1970s
Angioplasty	1978
Thrombolytics[b]	1980s

Source: Prospective Payment Assessment Commission, Medicare and the American Health Care System series, various issues.

a. The year of innovation refers to initial development. Other advances were made later.

b. Developed in the 1970s but not applied in heart attack care until the 1980s.

varied over time. Examinations of mortality reductions between 1950 and 1970 typically place a large role on primary and secondary prevention.[6] This was the time of the surgeon general's first report on the dangers of smoking (1965), so primary and secondary prevention would naturally have a large role to play in this period. Studies of more recent years have attributed a larger role to medical interventions. Between 1980 and 1990, for example, Hunink and others estimate that 43 percent of mortality reductions resulted from acute disease management.[7]

But the debate on this issue is not settled. Aggregate trends in cardiovascular disease health are difficult to interpret. Furthermore, it is particularly difficult to answer the subsequent questions that we want to ask, such as the cost-benefit analysis of medical interventions. To consider these factors, we focus on one type of cardiovascular illness in detail: the treatment of heart attacks.

The Efficacy of Heart Attack Treatment

We focus on heart attacks for several reasons: (1) they are perhaps the most severe manifestation of cardiovascular disease, so that mortality after a heart attack is quite important; (2) they are expensive, leading to questions about what we are getting for our money; (3) they are common; and (4) people with a heart attack will necessarily be admitted to a hospital, so that data on heart attack treatments and costs are easier to obtain than data on treatments and costs for many other conditions.[8]

6. Goldman and Cook (1984).

7. Hunink and others (1997).

8. The analysis of this section draws heavily on Heidenreich and McClellan (1997).

Heart attack mortality has fallen substantially over time. In 1975, according to death records maintained by the National Center for Health Statistics, heart attacks caused approximately 325,000 deaths. By 1995 that figure was down to 218,000, a reduction of almost one-third.[9] According to the National Hospital Discharge Survey and other data, approximately 454,000 hospitalizations for heart attacks occurred in 1975, increasing to approximately 590,000 heart attacks in 1995.[10] But the in-hospital mortality rate declined from 22 to 12.5 percent. This decline in deaths also corresponds to a mortality decline of approximately 30 percent.[11] We are interested in explaining what factors account for such rapid reductions in heart attack mortality in the presence of rather modest changes in heart attack incidence.

To measure changes in the treatment of heart attacks over time, we compiled results from the universe of clinical studies published in the medical literature. The field is enormous; we reviewed literally hundreds of published studies and meta-analyses of heart attack treatments and their effectiveness. We divide our review into changes in heart attack patient characteristics, changes in the acute treatment of heart attacks, and changes in other components of medical therapy (including prehospital care and secondary prevention). Because far more complete data are available on acute management than on other components of heart attack care, we analyze the consequences of these treatment changes in detail.

Changes in Heart Attack Patient Characteristics

Several population studies suggest little change between 1975 and 1995 in the characteristics of heart attack patients that might lead to mortality differences. The average age of AMI patients in the Minnesota and Worcester registries and the proportions of male and female patients were essentially constant. Slightly more patients have been diagnosed with shock at the time of AMI presentation (7.5 percent in 1975 versus 9 percent in 1988 in the Worcester population), suggesting increased mor-

9. National Center for Health Statistics (1979, 1997).

10. This increase resulted primarily from demographic changes associated with population growth and aging. According to NCHS, the incidence rate of heart attacks increased only slightly (from 0.21 to 0.22 percent).

11. Note that the number of in-hospital AMI deaths (around 100,000 in 1975, and around 70,000 in 1995) is substantially smaller than the total number of AMI deaths. The discrepancy is due to deaths occurring before hospitalization and deaths after discharge. But both sources of information on AMI mortality give a similar picture of substantial improvement.

tality risk. On the other hand, the proportion of certain types of heart attacks, which are also associated with higher mortality, appears to have declined, and the proportion of other types of heart attacks, ones that are associated with lower acute mortality, has increased. This latter change may well be a consequence of more effective acute restoration of blood flow. Finally, significantly fewer patients have high blood pressure at the time of their AMI, which may also be associated with lower mortality. Together, these factors suggest that average AMI case severity decreased slightly, potentially accounting for 10–20 percent of the decline in the average AMI mortality rate. Note that we do not attempt to distinguish the role of behavioral factors versus medical therapies like antihypertensive medications in accounting for these modest improvements. Their collective effects appear to be quite modest.

Changes in Acute Treatments

Table 2-5 shows summary results of the share of heart attack patients receiving a range of acute treatments (that is, treatments during or soon after the initial heart attack hospitalization) from the mid-1970s to the mid-1990s. The upper panel of the table shows data on pharmaceutical treatments, which have changed substantially over this time period. Thrombolytics, for example, were not used in heart attack care in 1980 but were used in almost one-third of heart attacks by 1995. The use of aspirin, beta blockers, and heparin also increased. Calcium-channel blocker use increased rapidly in the early 1980s and then fell, following the publication of studies documenting potentially harmful effects of their use in acute management. Use of lidocaine and other anti-arrhythmic agents also fell over the time period, in conjunction with new information on their potential harmfulness for typical AMI patients.

As the bottom panel of the table shows, substantial increases also occurred in the use of surgical interventions such as angioplasty (percutaneous transluminal coronary angioplasty, or PTCA), coronary artery bypass graft (CABG), and cardiac catheterization. For example, cardiac catheterization was performed acutely on 3 percent of heart attack patients in 1975 but on over 40 percent of heart attack patients in 1995.

The table demonstrates that even technologies that were well known in the mid-1970s diffused widely over the subsequent two decades. Comparing tables 2-3, 2-4, and 2-5, for example, shows that even though beta blockers were developed in the 1960s, their use more than doubled between the mid-1970s and mid-1990s. Changes in the perceived effec-

Table 2-5. *Use of Acute Interventions for Myocardial Infarction*[a]

Percent

Therapy	1973–77	1978–82	1983–87	1988–92	1993–96
Pharmaceuticals					
Beta blockers	20.6	41.5	47.5	47.3	48.8
Aspirin	15.0	14.1	20.1	62.0	75.0
Nitrates	55.8	83.1	93.2	n.a.	n.a.
Intravenous nitroglycerin	29.1[b]	40.9	76.4	n.a.	59.0
Heparin/anticoagulants	n.a.	n.a.	53.0	75.0	70.0
Calcium-channel blockers	0	0	63.9	59.0	31.0
Lidocaine	30.0	48.2	46.5	n.a.	16.2
Other anti-arrthymics	30.7	22.5	21.9	n.a.	n.a.
Magnesium	n.a.	n.a.	n.a.	n.a.	8.5
ACE inhibitors	0	n.a.	n.a.	n.a.	56.0
Thrombolytics	0	0	9.3	24.5	30.6
Procedures					
Catheterization	3.1	5.2	9.8	34.9	42.0
Primary angioplasty	0	0	0	n.a.	9.1
Any angioplasty	0	0	5.6	21.0	15.0
Coronary bypass	2.85[b]	5.7	8.0	10.0	9.5

Source: Based on literature review in Heidenreich and McClellan (1997).

n.a. Not available.

a. In-hospital or thirty-day use.

b. Average of 1970 and 1979 values.

tiveness of these technologies, new literature on actual effectiveness, and other changes in the medical environment clearly resulted in substantial changes in medical practice.

We also reviewed the medical literature to estimate the effect of these various interventions on acute AMI mortality (mortality within the first thirty days of a heart attack). Table 2-6 reports the estimated effects on relative mortality, along with confidence intervals, summarized from a variety of clinical trials and meta-analyses. Virtually all studies reported relative risk reductions (odds ratios) on case fatality rates—that is, the ratio of survival rates for people receiving that treatment to survival rates for people not receiving the treatment. Table 2-7 shows our estimates of the absolute mortality benefits of the changes in use of these technologies, extrapolated from their reported relative risk effects.[12]

12. We standardized the reported rates to thirty-day mortality effects by applying the relative mortality reductions reported in the studies to population estimates of a baseline thirty-day mortality rate in patients hospitalized with AMI of 22 percent (the 1975 case-fatality estimate for hospitalized AMI patients).

Table 2-6. *Effects of Acute Interventions on Acute Mortality after Myocardial Infarction*[a]

Percent

Pharmaceutical therapy	Odds ratio	Upper	Lower
Beta blockers	0.88	0.80	0.98
Aspirin	0.77	0.70	0.89
Nitrates	0.94	0.90	0.99
Heparin/anticoagulants	0.78	0.65	0.92
Calcium-channel blockers	1.12	0.92	1.39
Lidocaine	1.38	0.98	1.95
Magnesium	1.02	0.44	1.08
ACE inhibitors	0.94	0.89	0.98
Thrombolytics	0.75	0.71	0.79

Source: Data are based on literature review in Heidenreich and McClellan (1997).

a. The table reports effects on mortality risk reduction, that is, estimates greater than one for relative risk imply reductions in risk.

A number of caveats apply to our results. First, most of the trials were conducted in middle-aged males without very serious co-morbid diseases, so generalizing to all AMI patients requires some assumptions about the effects of treatment in other populations. Some evidence from a few trials among the elderly shows that effects may actually be larger for this group, mainly because the baseline mortality rates are higher. Our "best-guess" estimates assume proportional effects in all AMI patients. Second, physician acumen in allocating treatments to particular patients and determining the appropriate timing of interventions may also play an important role in the effectiveness of care. We do not account for improvements in acumen over time, but it is likely that accumulating experience with the technologies would increase their effectiveness. Third, as technologies diffuse more widely, they could be used in more "marginal" cases, where benefits are smaller.[13] This effect may offset the experience effect, but again there is no easy way to quantify its magnitude. Finally, not all trials of particular treatments were conducted with a particular pattern of use of all the other treatments. For example, one might expect a smaller effect of heparin (which reduces blood clotting) in patients who are also receiving aspirin (which also limits blood clotting). In deriving our population estimates and ranges, we have tried to take such interactions into account, based on empirical evidence where it is available and based on reasonable clinical considerations otherwise. The

13. McClellan (1996).

Table 2-7. *Estimated Acute Mortality Benefits of Changes in Acute Treatment of Heart Attack*

Therapy	Absolute benefit[a]	Adjusted benefit[b]	Change in use, 1975–95 (percent)	Share of mortality reduction explained (percent)[c]			
				Estimate 1	Estimate 2	Upper	Lower
Pharmaceuticals							
Beta blockers	0.021	0.018	239	5	5	9	1
Aspirin	0.042	0.038	60	23	23	30	11
Nitrates	0.010	0.008	30	0	3	5	0
Heparin/anticoagulants	0.040	0.008	4	0	1	2	0
Calcium-channel blockers	−0.020	−0.015	31	0	−2	3	−5
Lidocaine	−0.060	−0.045	−15	0	7	0	0
Magnesium	−0.003	−0.003	8.5	0	0	7	0
ACE inhibitors	0.010	0.008	24	2	2	3	1
Thrombolytics	0.045	0.036	31	11	11	13	9
Procedures							
Primary angioplasty	0.045	0.036	9.1	3	3	4	3
Other angioplasty	0.010	0.008	15	0	1	6	0
Coronary bypass	0.010	0.008	6.7	0	1	3	0
Total				45	55	85	20

Source: Based on data analysis in Heidenreich and McClellan (1997).

a. Based on meta-analysis odds ratio and 1975 mortality of 22 percent.

b. Adjusted for interactions between therapies.

c. Percent of 1975–95 decrease in heart attack case fatality rates explained by changes in use of each treatment. Estimate 1 assumes mortality effect for only beta-blockade, aspirin, thrombolytics, ACE inhibition, and primary angioplasty. Estimate 2 assumes that the true benefit or harm for each drug equals the estimate from meta-analysis. "Upper" uses the favorable 95 percent confidence limit of the mortality reduction for each drug. "Lower" uses the unfavorable 95 percent confidence limit and assumes that only aspirin, primary angioplasty, thrombolytics, and ACE inhibitors affect mortality.

resulting "adjusted" estimates of the acute mortality benefit are reported in the third column of table 2-7.[14]

The fourth column of table 2-7 reports the change in use rates (in percentage points) for each of the technologies. The remainder of the table reports shares of acute mortality improvements explained by changes in the use of each treatment.

All of the estimated shares are based on our adjusted benefit estimates. The share calculations are based on a total reduction in acute mortality from 22 to 12 percent. In other words, if survival conditional on hospitalization with a heart attack had not changed between 1975 and 1995, approximately 30,000 more heart attack patients would have died in 1995. In attributing the mortality reduction to particular treatments, estimate 1 in table 2-7 assumes that only five of the technologies studied have nonzero mortality effects: beta blockers, aspirin, thrombolytics, ACE inhibitors, and primary PTCA.[15] The clinical trial evidence on the effects of these treatments is strong, so this is our most conservative "best estimate." Estimate 2 includes our best estimates of the effects of the other technologies, based on somewhat weaker and unsettled clinical evidence. Finally, the "upper" and "lower" estimates provide extreme bounds on the estimated effects of the treatment changes. They are based on the upper (most effective) and lower (least effective) 95 percent confidence limits on the estimated treatment effects reported in published meta-analyses.

Table 2-7 shows that three drug therapies—aspirin, thrombolytics, and beta blockers—resulted in the largest improvements in heart attack mortality. For example, beta blocker use increased from 20 to about 50 percent of AMI patients during this period. Based on our best estimate of the average reduction in acute mortality from beta blockers (1.8 percentage points), this change in AMI treatment accounted for approximately 5 percent of the total acute mortality reduction for heart attacks,

14. Some prior studies included treatment arms that allowed estimation of interaction effects of certain treatments (for example, beta blockers and thrombolytics). These studies generally have shown that the combined effects of the interventions we study have less than fully additive effects. Where such evidence is not available, we used clinical considerations about mechanisms of action. In particular, for our "best-guess" estimates, we assumed that the use of aspirin, beta blockers, and thrombolytics (key technologies for anticoagulation and forced increased blood flow to the heart) would lead to a 50 percent reduction in the effects of other technologies with similar mechanisms of action, if those effects were estimated in studies that did not use these treatments. The adjusted effect estimates account for this joint diffusion of technologies.

15. We assume that primary PTCA is used as an alternative to thrombolytics; in practice, relatively few patients receive both.

or approximately 1,500 fewer deaths in 1995. Similarly, the diffusion of thrombolytics resulted in approximately 3,300 fewer deaths, and aspirin (which became much more widely used between 1975 and 1995) resulted in approximately 6,900 fewer deaths. Some recent studies of calcium-channel blockers suggest that they increase mortality for AMI patients. Increased use of these drugs suggests a slightly higher mortality rate in 1995 over 1975, although the substantial decline in calcium-channel blocker use since 1985 has limited this effect. Increased use of cardiac procedures, in particular the diffusion of primary angioplasty as an alternative to thrombolytic drugs for reperfusion, also accounted for some of the mortality reduction.[16]

Taken together, our estimates imply that changes in the medical treatments used in the acute management of AMI account for approximately 55 percent of the reduction in mortality that has occurred in AMI cases between 1975 and 1995, with the bulk of this improvement (50 percent) coming from pharmaceuticals. If we restrict our analysis to the five technologies described above for which the evidence on treatment effects is strongest, we obtain a slightly smaller estimated share explained (45 percent, with 42 percent coming from pharmaceuticals). Even our most conservative estimates of the mortality improvement resulting from acute treatments suggest that they account for around 20 percent of the observed improvement in mortality.

The finding that procedure used has a relatively small effect on mortality improvements may understate the role of these technologies in contributing to mortality reductions. The estimates in table 2-7 do not account for any learning by doing. For example, if physicians get better at performing bypass surgery over time, the estimated effects of bypass surgery on outcomes should be increasing over time. Clinical studies do not capture learning-by-doing effects, however, so they are not incorporated into our table. Since learning by doing is much more important for intensive procedures than for pharmaceutical use (although there may be some for pharmaceuticals—for example, the best time to give the drug), we suspect this biases the results toward finding a lower share of mortality improvements resulting from intensive procedure use.

We also reviewed the more limited evidence on other sources of improvement in acute mortality over time. Though changes in monitor-

---

16. The estimated mortality effects of these procedures are limited; however, there is considerable evidence that they have had a larger incremental impact on the quality of life of AMI patients.

ing methods appear to have been relatively important sources of mortality improvements in the 1960s and early 1970s, coronary care units (CCUs) with close cardiac monitoring of heart attack patients had largely been diffused by the mid-1970s.[17] These CCU technologies support rapid detection and treatment of irregular heart rhythms and other serious complications. But because the vast majority of cardiac patients were being monitored by 1975, CCU monitoring has probably not played a major role in the acute mortality improvements since that time. The use of right-heart (pulmonary artery) catheterization for functional assessment in CCUs increased between 1975 and the late 1980s and then appears to have declined modestly after 1990. Use of these devices is controversial, and there is no clear evidence that they improve survival. Thus changes in cardiac monitoring probably did not result in any significant mortality improvements between 1975 and 1995.

Changes in Prehospital Care

Changes in prehospital care compose another potential source of acute mortality improvements. Though far fewer studies have been reported, they do not suggest that prehospital care has accounted for much of the improvement in acute mortality. For example, studies of 1975 and 1990 AMI patients have found similar rates of ambulance use and only modest increases in the availability of advanced cardiac life support (ACLS). Emergency 911 systems and (recently) enhanced 911 systems have become more widely available, and the content of ACLS procedures has evolved, but several studies have failed to document improvements in mortality following activation or enhancement of 911 systems. In the last several years, time between hospital arrival and the delivery of key AMI treatments (thrombolytics, primary angioplasty) appears to have declined. Reductions in "door to needle" time may reduce mortality; thrombolytic efficacy is linearly related to time between attack occurrence and drug treatment. But no reports exist on average times to reperfusion treatment. Taken together, it is likely that improvements in prehospital care and reductions in time to treatment have led to a modest improvement in AMI mortality, perhaps 5–10 percent, but this conclusion is speculative.

The factors we have described—changes in AMI patient characteristics, changes in acute treatment, and changes in prehospital care—appear to explain approximately 80 percent of the total improvement in acute

17. Goldman and Cook (1984).

mortality for heart attacks that occurred between 1975 and 1995. The remaining 20 percent may be the result of other technologies that we have not studied in detail, improvements in physician acumen in applying technologies, differential diffusion in subgroups of heart attack patients (with differential effects), and miscellaneous other factors. Within the 80 percent explained, acute treatments for AMI, and especially pharmaceutical treatments, are responsible for the bulk of the mortality reductions. Diffusion of invasive cardiac procedures, innovations in prehospital care, and more favorable characteristics of heart attack patients on admission have been responsible for small shares of the mortality improvements.

Post-Acute Treatment and Secondary Prevention

Published studies are also inadequate for more than speculative discussion of the factors responsible for improvements in post-acute mortality for heart attack patients. Because the complications of heart attacks—including heart failure and chronic ischemic damage to the heart muscle—are responsible for more deaths than heart attacks alone, the long-term improvements in mortality may be even more substantial than the acute improvements. Many innovations have occurred in the treatment of patients with substantial damage to their heart from the attacks, including expanded cardiac rehabilitation programs as well as drug therapies such as ACE inhibitors and anticoagulation therapy. The number of heart attack patients surviving with impaired function is clearly increasing, and these treatments have been shown to reduce mortality in patients with heart failure. However, few studies have quantified the effects of long-term therapies for heart failure patients. The best evidence exists for ACE inhibitors, but limited quantitative data on the changes in heart failure prevalence after heart attacks make it difficult to quantify these important effects.

The same is true about secondary prevention of AMI through diagnostic procedures for risk stratification, risk factor counseling, pharmacologic therapies, and invasive procedures. Once again, studies show that many of these techniques result in significant reductions in long-term mortality after heart attacks, but we do not have data on changes in utilization or efficacy of these therapies for populations of heart attack survivors. Furthermore, it is likely that these treatments have important interactions with the changes in acute treatment of AMI. For example, AMI patients are now more likely to have blood flow to the heart restored acutely through thrombolytic drugs or primary angioplasty and are less likely to have subsequent blockages develop in the same or different coronary blood vessels because of cholesterol-lowering drugs and aspirin.

The factors discussed here suggest that innovations in primary prevention, acute and post-acute management, and secondary prevention have led to substantial reductions in acute and long-term AMI mortality. We cannot quantify each of the components of improved long-term health, but medical interventions appear to be particularly important. Among these medical interventions, increased use of some key pharmaceutical agents—particularly aspirin, thrombolytics, and beta blockers—has led to the largest reductions in heart attack mortality.

The Costs and Benefits of Heart Attack Care

Understanding the aggregate benefits of new technologies does not answer all of our questions.[18] We are also interested in the cost of these interventions and how the costs relate to the benefits. Since aggregate data cannot answer these questions, therefore, we use two more detailed sources of data.

The first data set is a complete record of detailed services, charges, demographic information, and discharge abstracts for all heart attack patients (patients discharged with a principal diagnosis of ICD-9 CM codes 410.00–410.99) admitted to one particular major teaching hospital (MTH) between 1983 and 1994. Each specific billable service that the hospital provided is reported in the data. We restrict the sample to those patients for whom the observed heart attack was their first at this hospital, roughly 300 episodes annually.[19]

The second source of data is Medicare claims records for all elderly patients with a heart attack between 1984 and 1991. These records contain much less detail on services received than do our hospital-specific service data; only major procedures and days in the hospital are reliably coded. However, the Medicare data have two important advantages relative to the MTH data. First, because Medicare is the primary payer for the vast majority of elderly Americans, we are able to construct comprehensive estimates of expenditures on medical care for almost all elderly AMI patients from 1984 to 1991, roughly 230,000 patients annually. We

18. The analysis in this section and the next draws heavily on Cutler and others (1998).

19. We do not know whether the patients had an earlier heart attack elsewhere. However, we do know whether or not they were transferred to MTH from another hospital. We have experimented with restricting the sample to nontransfers, without important effects on the results.

limit our analysis to hospital costs, since hospital costs compose the predominant expense in caring for AMI patients. Second, one can link Medicare data to Social Security death records and thereby determine survival outcomes.

We date the onset of the heart attack at the first admission to a hospital with a heart attack diagnosis—the box on the left in figure 2-3. As noted above, a person who suffers a heart attack will almost always be admitted to a hospital unless he or she dies before reaching one (in which case the cost of treatment is not very interesting) because the initial treatments for AMI must all be administered in an inpatient setting. While they survive, patients may receive care for their heart attack, in and out of hospitals, over the following months. For example, patients may receive tests or invasive diagnostic procedures in the initial hospital admission and be readmitted for additional tests or invasive procedures later on. We group all care received within ninety days of the initial heart attack in the same heart attack episode. All of our subsequent results are based on heart attack episodes.

We begin by examining the aggregate mortality experience of people suffering a heart attack from the Medicare data. Figure 2-4 shows cumulative mortality rates for the elderly for various time periods after a heart attack: one day, ninety days, and one through five years. Substantial reductions in mortality rates following a heart attack have occurred in the elderly. Mortality during the initial hospital stay fell nearly 2 percentage points. Mortality at one year fell by considerably more, 5 percentage points. Because the mortality data only extend through the end of 1992, we cannot measure mortality rates in 1991 for time periods longer than a year. Still, the data through 1987 suggest declines in cumulative mortality rates at periods beyond one year as well.[20]

As noted above, medical care may be only one factor in this mortality improvement: risk factor modification or environmental changes may also be important. One way to judge the importance of these factors, which affect all the elderly equally, is to consider increased life expectancy for people with heart attack compared to the overall elderly population. The difference will be a more accurate indicator of the benefits of

---

20. It is important to recognize that these changes represent changes in *average* health following a heart attack. A substantial amount of evidence suggests that the *marginal* amount of medical care—even care for heart attacks—provides benefits at relatively high cost (Cutler [1995]; Cutler and Staiger [1996]; McClellan [1996]; McClellan, McNeil, and Newhouse [1994]; McClellan and Newhouse [1997]; Newhouse and McClellan [1998]). For our work, we care about average health benefits, but in other circumstances we might be more concerned about marginal benefits.

Figure 2-4. *Cumulative Mortality Rate Following a Hospitalization*

Cumulative mortality rate (percent)

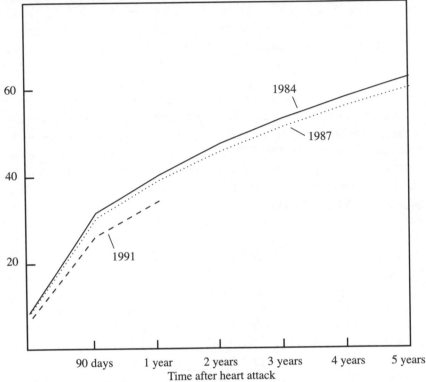

Time after heart attack

Source: Authors' calculations.

medical care than the reduction in heart attack mortality alone.[21] When
we do this comparison, we find the overall elderly population's life expectancy increased only by four months, or half as long. Thus medical care
likely has some effects on heart attack survival.

The fact that mortality has been falling after a heart attack confirms
the evidence from the medical literature. The fact that mortality has been
falling so rapidly in the first day after the heart attack strongly implies

21. This methodology is not exact. Reductions in aggregate mortality resulting from some
factors (for example, better control of blood sugar for diabetics) will reduce mortality for heart
attack sufferers more than mortality for the general population, whereas reductions in aggregate
mortality from other factors (for example, better cancer therapy) will have a smaller effect on
heart attack patients than the general population. In both of these cases, the difference in
mortality reductions between heart attack patients and the overall population will include more
than just the effect of heart attack treatments, but the sign of the bias is unknown.

that the set of early interventions—thrombolytic therapies, better 911 systems, improved EMT care—have had a particularly large effect on mortality. This again confirms our findings from the medical literature.

Increased Survival after a Heart Attack

To examine the importance of these mortality reductions for overall health of people with an AMI, we turn them into an increase in life expectancy after a heart attack. Estimating life expectancy from mortality rates is not trivial; a number of imputations are involved.[22] In the interest of brevity, we omit the details here.

The first column of table 2-8 shows life expectancy after a heart attack. In 1984 the average person with a heart attack lived five years and two months. By 1991 the average heart attack sufferer lived five years and ten months, an increase of eight months.

The benefits of heart attack treatments might show up in improved quality of life as well as length of life, but morbidity after a heart attack is difficult to measure. Few studies have evaluated the detailed functional capabilities of people with a heart attack over time.[23] For instance, can people walk up a flight of stairs without pain? We thus stick with the mortality benefits of changes in heart attack therapies. Since table 2-2 showed that morbidity for heart attack survivors was likely improving over time, this should bias us toward understating the full benefits of heart attack treatments.

The Costs of AMI Treatment

In addition to estimating the benefits of heart attack care, we can also estimate its costs. Figure 2-5 shows the average cost of treating a heart attack between 1984 and 1991, based on the Medicare data. The third and fourth columns of table 2-8 show the level and cumulative change in costs over time. We report costs in 1991 dollars (adjusted using the GDP deflator). The cost of a heart attack has increased from about $11,000 in 1984 to about $15,000 in 1991, for a real increase of 4 percent annually.

Table 2-9 shows more information on these costs. The first row shows total hospital spending on heart attacks. Heart attack spending increased from $2.6 billion in 1984 (in 1991 dollars) to $3.4 billion in 1991. The

22. Cutler and others (1998) discuss this in more detail.
23. See Cutler and Richardson (1997) for one such attempt.

Table 2-8. *Life Expectancy and Cost Following a Heart Attack*[a]

Year	Heart attack population				Overall elderly population				Net change (heart attack — overall elderly)	
	Life expectancy (years)	Change in life value (dollars)	Costs (dollars)	Change in costs (dollars)	Life expectancy (years)	Change in life value (dollars)	Costs (dollars)	Change in costs (dollars)	Change in life value (dollars)	Change in costs (dollars)
1984	5 2/12	...	11,123	...	10 3/12	...	1,667	...	...	...
1985	5 4/12	2,821	11,638	514	10 2/12	–823	1,768	100	3,644	414
1986	5 4/12	3,277	11,980	856	10 3/12	369	1,779	112	2,907	745
1987	5 5/12	5,180	12,250	1,127	10 4/12	1,430	1,791	124	3,750	1,003
1988	5 6/12	7,799	12,746	1,622	10 3/12	–86	1,865	198	7,885	1,425
1989	5 8/12	10,899	13,076	1,953	10 5/12	3,186	1,936	268	7,703	1,685
1990	5 9/12	13,637	13,681	2,558	10 6/12	5,022	1,945	278	8,614	2,280
1991	5 10/12	14,860	14,851	3,727	10 7/12	6,530	2,080	412	8,330	3,315

Source: Authors' calculations.

a. The sample is all elderly Medicare beneficiaries with a new heart attack. Costs are in 1991 dollars.

Figure 2-5. *Medicare Reimbursement per Heart Attack, 1984–91*

Average reimbursement per heart attack (1991 dolllars)

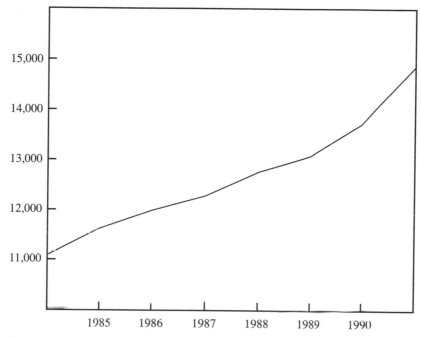

Source: Authors' calculations.

second row shows the incidence of heart attacks in the Medicare data. Heart attack incidence has actually been falling over time, in part because of improved primary and secondary prevention. As a result, cost per heart attack, shown in the third row of the table, has been increasing even more rapidly than total heart attack costs.[24]

What can explain this increasing cost of heart attack care? Table 2-9 shows Medicare reimbursement for our different treatment regimens over time. Reimbursement conditional on a treatment regimen was relatively constant or even falling in real terms over this period. This is particularly true for angioplasty, for which reimbursement fell 6 percent annually. This large reduction was by design; angioplasty reimbursement was reduced in 1986 as Medicare administrators cut payments to more

24. The numbers in table 2-9 do not match those in table 2-8 precisely because the data in table 2-8 are adjusted for the average demographic mix of the heart attack population over the 1984–91 period, whereas the numbers in table 2-9 use the population of heart attack patients that year. As a comparison of the tables indicates, the demographic adjustment is relatively unimportant.

Table 2-9. *Technological Change and Expenditures in Cardiac Procedure Use, 1984–91*

Treatment	Intensive procedure use[a] (percent)			Average hospital reimbursement[a]		
	1984	1991	Annual change[b]	1984 (dollars)	1991 (dollars)	Annual change (percent)
Total spending	n.a.	n.a.	n.a.	2.6 billion	3.4 billion	3.9
Number of patients	n.a.	n.a.	n.a.	233,295	227,182	−0.3
Average reimbursement	n.a.	n.a.	n.a.	11,175	14,772	4.0
Medicare						
Medical management	88.7	59.4	−4.2	9,829	10,783	1.3
Catheterization only	5.5	15.5	1.4	15,380	13,716	−1.6
Angioplasty	0.9	12.0	1.6	25,841	17,040	−5.9
Bypass surgery	4.9	13.0	1.2	28,135	32,117	1.9
Major teaching hospital						
Medical management	65.0	23.0	−4.7	13,900[c]	11,769	−1.8
Catheterization only	20.0	21.0	0.1	15,290	15,105	−0.1
Angioplasty	3.0	30.0	3.0	16,124	18,441	1.5
Bypass surgery	11.0	27.0	1.8	37,437	50,874	3.4

Source: Authors' calculations.

n.a. Not available.

a. Costs are in 1991 dollars adjusted using the GDP deflator.

b. Growth is average percentage point change each year.

c. Costs for major teaching hospital are an average of 1983–85 and 1992–94.

accurately reflect the estimated cost of performing the treatment. Catheterization-only payments were also reduced, as more catheterizations were performed during the initial hospital stay rather than on a subsequent admission. Reimbursement for medically managed heart attacks or bypass surgery increased marginally.[25] The MTH accounting cost data, shown in the last rows of the table, generally exhibit the same pattern, although these data include the non-Medicare population as well. Thus price increases per type of service received do not appear to explain the growth of spending.

In contrast to the relatively flat prices for given therapies, there has been a dramatic increase in the use of more intensive therapies over time. Figure 2-6 shows the use of intensive surgical therapy for heart attack patients in the Medicare data. Use of cardiac catheterization rose from 10 percent in 1984 to over 40 percent by 1991. Bypass surgery rates increased from 5 to 15 percent, and angioplasty rates went from 1 to 15 percent.

Because Medicare pays more for more intensive care than for less intensive care, the increase in the intensity of medical treatment has had large effects on medical spending. Indeed, our data suggest that all of the growth of costs for heart attack treatment can be explained by the increase in the intensity of treatment, rather than by an increase in the cost of a standard type of care.

Cost-Benefit Analysis of Heart Attack Treatment

To compare the costs and benefits of heart attack treatment, we need a dollar value for a year of life. Estimating the worth of a life is very controversial.[26] We use as a central estimate a value per life-year of $25,000. This estimate is low compared to others in the literature; for example, George Tolley, Donald Kenkel, and Robert Fabian suggest a value per life-year of $75,000–150,000.[27] Thus we are likely to find less beneficial care than others would suggest. The second column of table 2-8 shows the change in the value of health for heart attack survivors implied by this estimate. Between 1984 and 1991, the value of additional life increased by nearly $15,000. Comparing the second and fourth columns of table 2-8, we find that the increase in the value of additional life ($15,000 by 1991) is greater than the increase in costs of heart attack care ($4,000 by 1991). In other words, we are better off for having spent our

25. See Cutler and McClellan (1998) for more details.
26. Viscusi (1993).
27. Tolley, Kenkel, and Fabian (1994).

Figure 2-6. *Increases in the Use of Intensive Technology for Heart Attack Patients*

Percent of patients receiving treatment

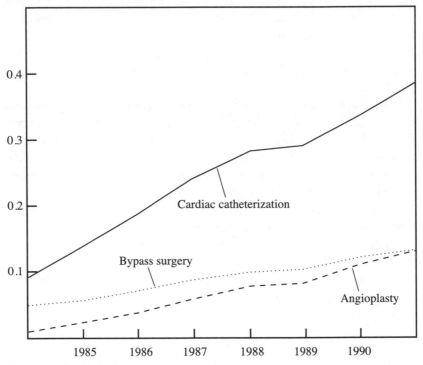

Source: Authors' calculations.

money on heart attack care than we would have been if the money had been spent elsewhere.

As noted above, comparing the heart attack population to the overall elderly population is one way to isolate the importance of heart attack—specific changes in treatments from overall changes in lifestyles, environments, or medical care as a whole. The middle columns of table 2-8 show similar changes in longevity and Medicare costs for the overall elderly population, matched to the demographic mix of the heart attack population. Life expectancy for people without a heart attack is (naturally) greater than life expectancy for people with a heart attack. In 1984, the average elderly person had a life expectancy of ten years and three months. Between 1984 and 1991, this increased by four months, to ten years and seven months. And there was a significant amount of increased Medicare spending associated with this—$412.

The last columns show the differential increase in longevity and Medicare costs for the heart attack population relative to the overall elderly population. The net improvement in length of life is still greater than the increase in treatment costs, although by a smaller amount. The health improvement was $11,000 greater than the increased costs using the heart attack population alone and $5,000 greater than the increased costs using the specification controlling for overall changes in the health of the elderly.

These results are extremely important; if they generalize to other medical treatments, they imply, for example, that the true "price" of medical care services has not been increasing nearly as rapidly as official indexes suggest.

Implications: A Price Index for Heart Attack Care

The finding of a positive benefit-cost difference for heart attack care implies that the real "price" of medical care has been falling over time. To see this, we need to discuss price indexes in somewhat more detail, distinguishing between two price indexes: the service price index and the cost-of-living index.[28]

The Service Price Index

The service price index is the index that was used in the past in the Bureau of Labor Statistics' CPI for medical care. Methodologically, this price index is constructed by choosing a fixed basket of goods and then pricing that same basket over time. We term this a service price index because it focuses on a given set of medical services, as opposed to the value to consumers of medical care.

For example, to calculate the hospital component of the CPI, the traditional Bureau of Labor Statistics' index priced charges for six hospital services at each hospital: two room services (for example, charges per day for semiprivate rooms and medical ICU rooms), three other inpatient services (for example, operating room time or electrocardiograms), and one outpatient service (for example, outpatient electrocardiogram). These services are then aggregated into a hospital index.[29]

The first row of table 2-10 shows the growth of the real (relative to the GDP deflator) medical care CPI from 1983 to 1994. Over this time period,

28. For more discussion of appropriate price indexes for medical care, see Shapiro and Wilcox (1996) and Triplett (1998).

29. See, for example, Bureau of Labor Statistics (1992) and Ford and Sturm (1988).

Table 2-10. *Summary of Price Indexes*

Percent

Index	Real annual change
Service price indexes[a]	
1. Medical care CPI	3.4
2. Synthetic CPI for MTH—charges	3.3
3. Synthetic CPI for MTH—costs	2.4
4. Annually rebased price index	0.7
5. Treatment regimen price index	0.4 to 0.6
Cost-of-living index	−1.1 to −0.5

Source: Authors' calculations.

a. Service price indexes are for the 1983–94 period, with the exception of treatment regimen price index for Medicare data (1984–91) and cost-of-living index (1984–91). Growth of price indexes is relative to the GDP deflator.

the real medical CPI rose by 3.4 percent annually. In the next row, we replicate this analysis using heart attack treatments at MTH. The real CPI for heart attacks at MTH grew at an annual rate of 3.3 percent, almost the same as the overall medical care CPI.

Very few payers pay charges (or list prices) for medical care. Discounts from charges are the norm, especially for hospital care, and the pricing of medical care needs to account for this.[30] To adjust for this factor, we formed an alternative price index based on the cost of medical care in MTH, rather than its charge. For the average payer, costs are more likely to be an accurate reflection of average prices than will charges. As the next row shows, a CPI based on costs instead of charges grew about a percentage point less each year, for an annual increase of 2.4 percent.

The traditional medical care CPI does not change the quantity of goods that are priced over time. For example, the hospital room component always priced the cost of one day in a hospital, independent of how long patients actually stay in the hospital. A more accurate price index would price the basket of goods that a typical patient is actually receiving over time. Then, as some services are substituted for other services, the price index would reflect that substitution. The next row of table 2-10 shows the growth of such a price index. We reweight the basket of goods that is provided annually. The growth of the index is much lower in this case, only 0.7 percent per year.

The final issue in the service price index is whether we want to price itemized medical services or whether we would rather price a more aggre-

30. Until recently, the Bureau of Labor Statistics was not able to account for this.

gated "treatment regimen," as in figure 2-2. Pricing treatment regimens may be more relevant than pricing a particular bundle of services; after all, it is much more natural to think that producers are supplying "bypass surgery at the current standard" than the particulars of surgery in any year. The next row of table 2-10 shows the price index based on treatment regimens. We can form this index using either the MTH data or the Medicare data. In both cases, the results are similar; the price index increases about 0.5 percent per year. The difference between this estimate and the official growth of the CPI is large; while the current CPI is increasing nearly 3.5 percent per year, our preferred service price index is increasing only 0.5 percent per year relative to the overall GDP deflator.

The Bureau of Labor Statistics has recently revised the CPI along the lines of our treatment regimen price index. The change was in part because many payers now reimburse medical care at the level of treatment regimens and in part because it was perceived to be a more accurate basis for pricing. This change in the CPI index may have important effects on measured inflation in the medical sector.

The Cost-of-Living Index

An alternative price index to the service price index is the cost-of-living index. Where the service price index asks about the cost of goods sold, the cost-of-living index asks about changes in the price of what consumers receive. The major difference between these two indexes is medical care quality. A higher quality bypass surgery operation may cost the same to produce but would be worth more to consumers. This additional value is an effective price reduction to consumers.

Formally, we define the change in the cost-of-living index as the increased spending on medical care over time less the additional value of that care. If medical care increases in cost without much improvement in health, that would be an increase in the cost of living. If medical care increases in cost but the value of that care rises over time, the cost-of-living index would be falling.[31]

The key to forming this index is to note that the cost and benefit of medical care are exactly what we calculated in the previous section. There

---

31. Formally, the cost-of-living index is the change in the expenditure required to produce a given level of utility. We can reconstitute this into two parts: the additional resources required by the medical sector and the health benefits of medical care. In particular, the quality adjusted cost of medical services equals the increase in medical spending less the dollar value of the improved health. Measuring the change in the cost of living involves estimating these latter two terms.

we showed that the benefits of heart attack care were greater than its additional costs. The implication is that the cost-of-living index for heart attack care is actually falling over time, not rising. The last row of table 2-10 shows our calculation of the cost-of-living index. Using the data on heart attack patients only (without an adjustment for the national population), our estimate is that the cost of living fell by 1.1 percent annually over the 1984–91 period. This finding is a direct consequence of our positive benefit-cost differential. When we control for changes in longevity and treatment costs for the Medicare population as a whole, the change in the cost-of-living index is -0.5 percent per year—smaller but still negative.

This calculation is striking.[32] Where current price indexes for medical care are increasing by 3–4 percent per year above general inflation, our best estimate of a quality-adjusted price index is falling by about 0.5–1 percent per year. Even if we ignore quality improvements, our preferred estimate of the price of heart attack treatments is that they are rising by perhaps 0.5 percent per year relative to other prices in the economy.

Managed Care and the Treatment of Heart Attacks

The final issue we explore is the effect of managed care on the treatment of heart attacks and on the benefit-cost analysis of the previous sections.[33] The $1 trillion American health care services industry is rapidly changing its structure. Traditionally, the provision of medical services and the payment for those services were separate industries. Patients and providers decided on appropriate treatments and insurers paid the bill. Increasingly, however, medical services and insurance are becoming integrated and care is being more regularly "managed." Insurers commonly use financial incentives to limit use, place restrictions on the services that may be provided, and form restrictive networks to bargain for lower prices from providers. Managed care has become the norm among the privately insured population. Whereas only one-quarter of the privately insured population was in managed care in 1987, three-quarters are enrolled in managed care today.[34]

In principle, managed care may be good or bad for heart attack treatments. While much popular discussion has focused on the potential for managed care to limit expensive treatments, it may also be the case that by

32. For additional empirical applications, see chapters 3 and 4, this volume; Cockburn (1997); Griliches and Cockburn (1994); and Shapiro and Wilcox (1996).
33. The analysis in this section draws heavily on Cutler, McClellan, and Newhouse (1998).
34. Gabel and others (1989); Jensen and others (1997).

getting people into the medical care system earlier, managed care increases the use of some technologies. It might also reduce the cost of the same medical care treatments. Ultimately, this is an empirical question.

We use two sources of data to examine the impact of managed care on heart attack treatment. The first is the complete claims records of a large firm in the Massachusetts area for the thirty months from July 1993 through December 1995 (the "firm data"). The firm has about 200,000 covered lives in its nonretiree population. It offers a traditional indemnity policy, a preferred provider organization (PPO), and several health management organizations (HMOs), which we generally group together. There are about 70,000–100,000 people in the indemnity and HMO policies, and about one-quarter that number in the PPO. For each plan, we know inpatient, outpatient, and prescription drug spending for all enrollees. We also know major procedures provided. We can thus look at total spending by plan and the use of particular forms of care.

Our second source of data is the complete set of inpatient claims for people admitted to hospitals in Massachusetts in fiscal years 1994 and 1995 (the "state data"). Beginning with calendar year 1994, hospitals provided social security numbers for the patients they admitted, so that admissions can be linked (even across hospitals) to form an episode of care. In the state data, we have several thousand heart attack episodes in indemnity policies, PPOs, and HMOs. The state data have more heart attack patients than the firm data, so they are better for analyzing the relation between type of insurance and inpatient care received. The state data do not contain reimbursement information, however, so we cannot look at spending differences with these data.

To examine differences in spending on heart attacks, we form ninety-day episodes of heart attack treatment, in the same fashion as our previous analysis. The upper panel of table 2-11 shows summary statistics on reimbursement for heart attacks using the firm data. The first column shows average reimbursement for all patients. Heart attacks are expensive; average reimbursement in the indemnity policy is $38,501 in the first ninety days. Reimbursement is much lower in the other plans. Average reimbursement in the PPO is only 69 percent as high as in the indemnity policy ($26,483), and only 61 percent as high ($23,631) in the HMO.

The next four columns of table 2-11 show reimbursement and the share of patients by treatment regimen.[35] Reimbursement differences

_____

35. We do not show statistics for the PPO because the number of heart attack patients is so small.

Table 2-11. *Heart Attack Reimbursement and Treatment, by Plan*

U.S. Dollars, unless otherwise specified

Plan	Average reimbursement (unadjusted)	Treatment regimen					Average reimbursement (adjusted)
		Medical management	Cardiac catheterization	Bypass surgery	Angioplasty		
Average reimbursement[a]							
Indemnity	38,501	24,720	47,105	106,302	44,542		40,329
Blue Cross/Blue Shield as preferred							
provider	26,483	n.a.	n.a.	n.a.	n.a.		n.a.
HMO	23,632	14,475	24,447	55,826	24,097		22,048
HMO as percent of indemnity	61	59	52	53	54		55
Treatment shares—firm data (percent)							
Indemnity	n.a.	56	23	7	13		n.a.
HMO	n.a.	53	16	14	17		n.a.
Treatment shares—state data (percent)							
Blue Cross/Blue Shield and indemnity	n.a.	41	19	14	26		n.a.
Non-HMO managed care	n.a.	35	21	16	27		n.a.
HMO	n.a.	44	17	14	25		n.a.

Source: Authors' calculations.

n.a. Not available

a. Reimbursement is within ninety days of the initial heart attack.

within treatment regimens mirror the overall reimbursement differences. In each case, reimbursement in the HMOs is only 50–60 percent as high as reimbursement in the indemnity policy. In contrast, the share of patients receiving different treatment regimens is roughly the same in the different plans. In the firm data, managed care patients are slightly *more* likely to receive intensive surgical procedures than are patients in the indemnity insurance policy; in the state data, managed care patients are slightly less likely to receive intensive surgical procedures than are patients in indemnity insurance. The final column of table 2-11 shows that adjusted for differences in the share of patients receiving different treatments, reimbursement in the HMOs is still only 55 percent of reimbursement in the indemnity policy.

Thus it appears that essentially all of the cost differences across plans result from differences in reimbursement conditional on a treatment regimen rather than a different type of care provided. We formalize this finding in table 2-12, where we estimate regression models for treatments and reimbursement as a function of the type of insurance the individual is enrolled in. We also include several control variables, including five-year age dummy variables, a dummy variable for men, dummy variables for region in the state, and the logarithm of median household income in the person's zip code, taken from the 1990 census.[36]

The first two columns show ordinary least squares estimates of the probability that a patient receives cardiac catheterization or coronary revascularization.[37] Men are more likely to receive intensive treatment than are women. Income is not related to treatment intensity, but people from MSAs are more likely to receive these procedures than are people outside of MSAs (not reported). The insurance variables are similar to the means in table 2-11. Controlling for demographics, HMO patients are a bit less likely to receive intensive procedures than are patients in indemnity insurance. This effect is statistically significant for catheterization but not for revascularization. The magnitude of these effects is relatively small, however—about 2–3 percentage points.

The third column of the table shows the effect of insurance on reimbursement conditional on the treatment regimen. In contrast to the re-

---

36. In the firm data, we divide people into those living in Boston, those living in another metropolitan statistical area (MSA), and those living outside of an MSA. In the state data, we include a dummy variable for different MSAs and a dummy variable for people living outside of an MSA.

37. We use ordinary least squares estimates to be compatible with our later instrumental variables estimates. Logit models of treatment regimens yield very similar results.

Table 2-12. *Estimates of the Effect of Insurance on Treatments and Reimbursement for Heart Attacks*[a]

Percent

| | State treatment data | | Firm data |
Variable	Cardiac catheterization	Coronary revascularization	ℓn (reimbursement)
Insurance			
HMO	−.034**	−.025	−.578**
	(.017)	(.017)	(.060)
Non-HMO managed	.018	−.008	n.a.
care	(.019)	(.020)	
Demographics			
Male	.039**	.053**	.057
	(.017)	(.017)	(.060)
White	−.132**	−.104**	n.a.
	(.025)	(.025)	
ℓn (median income)	.034	.037	.184*
	(.028)	(.029)	(.103)
Previous admission	.003	.000	.102*
	(.021)	(.022)	(.064)
Summary statistics			
N	4,243	4,243	853
σ_ε^2	.217	.226	.635

Source: Authors' calculations.

a. Care is all services provided within ninety days of the initial heart attack admission. All regressions include five year-age dummy variables and region dummy variables. Standard errors are in parentheses.

*Significant at 10 percent.

**Significant at 5 percent.

sults for treatment differences, we find large effects of insurance on reimbursement for a given treatment regimen. The coefficient on the HMO dummy variable implies that HMOs pay 44 percent less than indemnity insurance (exp[−.58]), and this is statistically significant.

The implication of these results is that essentially all of the difference between managed care and traditional insurance is on the prices paid for medical care, not the amount of medical care received.

Although this result is clear in our data, we want to be cautious on several grounds. First, the data are from only one state, and managed care is likely to differ across the country. Second, heart attacks probably involve less discretion in the choice of treatment than other diseases such as depression or common outpatient care. This is because managed care rarely provides its own heart attack treatment; it typically contracts with cardiologists and cardiovascular surgeons who also see patients not in managed care. Indeed, other studies show larger differences in the treatment of depression across insurance plans than we find here.[38] Finally, we suspect that the effect of managed care varies over time, so that more recent data could yield different conclusions than we found in our time period.

Conclusions

Our results suggest several important conclusions. First, although we pay more for medical care than we used to, we also get more in return. Both our review of the medical literature and our examination of medical records document a large role for medical care in improving the health of heart attack patients. In our sample of Medicare beneficiaries with a heart attack, we estimate that for an additional cost of $4,000 per heart attack patient, a patient's life may be extended by an average of eight months. Even at very modest estimates of the value per life-year, the additional spending on heart attacks has been worth the cost.

This conclusion has direct implications for productivity and price measurement in the medical sector. Receiving more in improved health than we pay in treatment costs implies that medical care is a more productive investment than the average use of our funds outside the medical sector. And it implies that a true cost-of-living index for heart attack care—a price index for health after a heart attack—is falling over time, whereas conventional medical care price indexes have suggested a rapid rise.

The important question is whether our results generalize to other types of medical care. We do not know the answer to this question. Heart attacks are clearly different from other conditions: they are acute, and they are very technologically intensive. In a medical care system accused of having a bias toward high-tech treatment of very severe illness, this suggests heart attacks may be a best-case analysis. On the other hand, there is a long-standing literature suggesting only a small role for acute interventions in improved cardiovascular disease health. The fact that we find such a large role for medical care in the treatment of a condition commonly believed to respond more to behavior than to medical inputs suggests that our findings might be indicative of the medical sector more broadly.

Perhaps most importantly, our results provide a framework for analyzing these issues in the future. Measuring the productivity of the medical

38. See chapter 3, this volume.

care sector—and the service sector more generally—has long been a problem in national income accounting. The methodology in this study suggests a way to tackle this fundamental issue. Along with other research on the price and output of the medical sector, this provides guidance for how to learn about these issues in the years to come.[39]

References

Braunwald, Eugene. 1997. *Heart Disease: A Textbook of Cardiovascular Medicine.* Saunders.

Bureau of Labor Statistics. 1992. "The Consumer Price Index." In *BLS Handbook of Methods*, bulletin 2414 (September).

Cockburn, Iain. 1997. "Price Indices for the Treatment of Arthritis." University of British Columbia.

Cutler, David M. 1995. "The Incidence of Adverse Medical Outcomes under Prospective Payment." *Econometrica* 63(1) (February): 29–50.

Cutler, David M., and Mark McClellan. 1998. "What Is Technological Change?" In *Inquiries in the Economics of Aging*, edited by David Wise, pp. 51–78. University of Chicago Press.

Cutler, David M., Mark McClellan, and Joseph Newhouse. 1998. "Prices and Productivity in Managed Care Insurance." Working Paper 6677. Cambridge: National Bureau of Economic Research.

Cutler, David M., and Elizabeth Richardson. 1997. "Measuring the Health of the United States Population." In *Brookings Papers on Economic Activity: Microeconomics,* pp. 217–71. Brookings Institution.

Cutler, David M., and Douglas Staiger. 1996. "Measuring the Value of Medical Progress." Harvard University.

Cutler, David M., and others. 1998. "Are Medical Prices Declining?" *Quarterly Journal of Economics* (November): 991–1024.

Ford, Ina Kay, and Philip Sturm. 1988. "CPI Revision Provides More Accuracy in the Medical Care Services Component." *Monthly Labor Review* 111 (April): 17–26.

Gabel, Jon, and others. 1989. "Employer-Sponsored Health Insurance in America." *Health Affairs* (Summer): 116–28.

Goldman, Lee, and E. Francis Cook. 1984. "The Decline in Ischemic Heart Disease Mortality Rates: An Analysis of the Comparative Effects of Medical Interventions and Changes in Lifestyle." *Annals of Internal Medicine* 101: 825–36.

Griliches, Zvi, and Iain Cockburn. 1994. "Generics and New Goods in Pharmaceutical Price Indexes." *American Economic Review* 84(5) (December): 1213–32.

Heidenreich, Paul, and Mark McClellan. 1998. "Trends in Heart Attack Treatments and Outcomes, 1975–1995: A Literature Review and Synthesis," in a volume edited by Ernst R. Berndt and David Cutler emanating from the Conference on Research in Income and Wealth (forthcoming).

Hunink, Maria G. M., and others. 1997. "The Recent Decline in Mortality from Coronary Heart Disease, 1980–1990: The Effect of Secular Trends in Risk Factors

39. Shapiro and Wilcox (1996); Triplett (1998); see also chapters 3 and 4, this volume.

and Treatment." *Journal of the American Medical Association* 277(7) (February 19): 535–42.

Isselbacher, Kurt, and others. 1994. *Harrison's Principles of Internal Medicine.* 13th ed. McGraw-Hill.

Jensen, Gail A., and others. 1997. "The New Dominance of Managed Care: Insurance Trends in the 1990s." *Health Affairs* (January/February): 125–36.

McClellan, Mark. 1996. "Changes in the Marginal Value of Medical Care." Stanford University.

McClellan, Mark, Barbara J. McNeil, and Joseph P. Newhouse. 1994. "Does More Intensive Treatment of Acute Myocardial Infarction Reduce Mortality?" *Journal of the American Medical Association* 272(11) (September 21): 859–66.

McClellan, Mark, and Joseph P. Newhouse. 1997. "The Marginal Costs and Benefits of Medical Technology." *Journal of Econometrics* 77: 39–64.

National Center for Health Statistics. 1979. *Vital Statistics of the United States, 1975: Volume II—Mortality, Part A.* Hyattsville, Md.

———. 1997. *Monthly Vital Statistics Report* 46(1) (September 11): 24, table 11.

Newhouse, Joseph P., and Mark McClellan. 1998. "Econometrics in Outcomes Research." *Annual Review of Public Health* 19: 17–34.

Shapiro, Matthew, and David Wilcox. 1996. "Mismeasurement in the Consumer Price Index." *NBER Macroeconomics Annual* 11: 93–142.

Tolley, George, Donald Kenkel, and Robert Fabian, eds. 1994. *Valuing Health for Policy: An Economic Approach.* University of Chicago Press.

Triplett, Jack E. 1998. "What's Different about Health? Human Repair and Car Repair in National Accounts." Paper presented at the Conference on Research in Income and Wealth's "Conference on Medical Care," Bethesda, Md., June 12–13, 1998.

Viscusi, W. Kip. 1993. "The Value of Risks to Life and Health." *Journal of Economic Literature* 31(4): 1912–46.

3

Price Indexes for the Treatment of Depression

Richard G. Frank, Ernst R. Berndt, and Susan H. Busch

T HE CONCEPTUAL FOUNDATIONS and interpretation of the Bureau of Labor Statistics (BLS) medical care price index have long been controversial. Echoing ideas discussed even earlier, Anne Scitovsky suggested that instead of collecting data on prices of selected medical care inputs such as physicians' fees for office visits, hospital room rates, and prescription drugs, as the BLS did at that time (and to some extent still does today), a preferable medical care price index would be based on the entire episodic treatment cost of selected illnesses or conditions, including any effects on changed medical outcomes.[1] Scitovsky concluded that it was feasible, albeit perhaps more costly, to implement a cost-per-episode-of-illness approach. Estimating the average costs of treatment in 1951–52 and 1964–65 for five specific illnesses or conditions using administrative records data from the Palo Alto Medical Research Foundation, Scitovsky found that the BLS price index rose considerably less rapidly than those based on her average-cost-of-treatment approach.[2]

We gratefully acknowledge research support from Eli Lilly and Company, the U.S. Bureau of Economic Analysis, National Science Foundation Grant SBR-9511550, and National Institute of Mental Health Grant MH43703. We are also grateful to Douglas Cocks, Thomas Croghan, M.D., David Cutler, Dennis Fixler, Mark McClellan, M.D., Will Manning, Thomas McGuire, Joseph Newhouse, and Jack Triplett for helpful comments on an earlier draft. Elizabeth Notman provided key programming support for this project.

1. See Gilbert (1961, 1962); Griliches (1962); Scitovsky (1967).
2. The BLS medical care price index rose about 59 percent from 1951 to 1965, whereas the percentage increases she found for acute appendicitis were 87 percent, maternity care 72 percent, otitis media in children 68 percent, cancer of the breast 106 percent, and fracture of the forearm from 55 to 315 percent (Scitovsky [1967], pp. 1183—84).

Three decades after Scitovsky's study, the U.S. Senate Finance Committee's Advisory Commission to Study the Consumer Price Index (1996) concluded that, by its best estimate, over the previous two decades the CPI overstated annual cost-of-living increases by about 1.1 percent overall and by 3.0 percent in several medical care categories.[3] Clearly the medical care marketplace in the 1990s is quite different from that in the 1950s and 1960s; now cost containment pressures are cutting back on laboratory and diagnostic testing, use of specialist physicians is being de-emphasized, and pressures from managed-care organizations are apparently bringing about greater discounts and physician price discrimination, even as health care policy analysts worry about possible deterioration in outcomes. The CPI Commission strongly endorsed a move in the CPI away from the pricing of health care inputs to an attempt to price medical care outcomes. It also recommended that the BLS develop and publish two separate cost-of-living indexes, one on a monthly basis and another annually, the latter incorporating more attention to quality issues and introducing improvements arising from new information and new research results.

Recent research has generated medical care price indexes that value health care outcomes rather than health care inputs for certain treatments and thereby begin to take quality change into account. Cutler and others, for example, contrast input price indexes for the cost of heart attack treatment, which rose by 6.7 percent over the period 1983–94, with an outcomes-adjusted index that takes into account a conservative valuation for the extension of life expectancy attributable to new heart attack treatments and increases by only 2.3 percent (in real terms, a decline of 1.1 percent) per year, implying a net upward bias of 4.4 percent per year.[4] Shapiro and Wilcox construct a price index for cataract surgery for the period 1969–93 and find that a CPI-like fixed-weight input-based index increases by a factor of about 9; a preferred alternative price index incorporating realized reduced levels of hospital services, but ignoring any improvements in the quality of medical outcomes, increases by only a factor of 3, implying an annual differential of 4.6 percent.[5]

In this chapter we build on the earlier work of Scitovsky, Cutler and others, and Shapiro and Wilcox in a number of ways. First, we consider a different category of illness, a mental health illness. Specifically, we focus on major depression, a prevalent and recurring illness associated with

3. U.S. Senate Finance Committee (1996), p. 60.
4. Cutler and others (1996).
5. Shapiro and Wilcox (1996).

widespread impairment and disability.[6] As in the case of other chronic illnesses, mortality is not a key endpoint, so outcomes may be more difficult to measure than in the case of, say, heart attacks. Second, we identify different service bundles for treating acute-phase depression that combine varying quantities of prescription drugs, medical management, and psychotherapy and then use transactions data to "price" these different bundles.

Third, we make use of results from clinical research to identify therapeutically similar treatment bundles that can then be linked and weighted to construct price indexes for treatment of specific forms of major depression. We employ various index number formulae that involve differing assumptions on the extent of ex ante substitutability among therapeutically similar treatment bundles. Because the medical community views treatment bundles as therapeutically similar in terms of efficacy, our linking of treatment bundles provides an important initial step toward incorporation of medical outcomes. Fourth, we distinguish a producer price index (PPI) representing the supply price or total receipts received by providers of the medical treatment (from insurers and patients) from the CPI, which incorporates the out-of-pocket costs (via copayments and deductible payments) by the patient-consumer. Finally, we present some initial price index calculations for the years 1991–95 that demonstrate the feasibility of implementing the approach and illustrate some striking differences in price movements for treatment of depression relative to the traditional medical CPI and PPI series.

Current BLS Procedures for the CPI and PPI

We begin with a brief overview of procedures and concepts currently employed by the BLS in its construction of CPI and PPI medical care price indexes.[7] In 1997 medical care accounted for about a 7.4 percent expenditure weight in the total CPI. Although total medical care expenditures as a percentage of GDP are about twice this weight, the medical care component of the CPI (the MCPI) weight reflects only a portion of total medical care outlays. Specifically, the MCPI weight reflects direct out-of-pocket cash outlays, household purchases of health insurance

6. See Greenberg and others (1993).
7. For more detailed discussion, albeit somewhat dated, see Getzen (1992); and Newhouse (1989).

(including Medicare Part B), plus employee contributions to health insurance premiums purchased through work. The MCPI excludes employer health insurance premium contributions, treating them as a business expense, and also excludes Medicare Part A as well as Medicaid outlays.[8]

The four major subindexes of the MCPI and their percentage weights within the aggregate MCPI are prescription drugs (12.1 percent), nonprescription drugs and medical supplies (5.3 percent), professional medical services (also called physicians' services, 47.1 percent), hospital and related services (30.7 percent), and health insurance (4.9 percent).[9] For each MCPI component, out-of-pocket payments plus the consumer-paid health insurance premium allocation yields a total component weight, which is then typically applied to prices paid by cash-paying customers; note that prices for many medical transactions could be quite different from cash prices, particularly in the last decade, as discounts to managed care organizations have become more common.[10]

Although planned changes have been announced and some are gradually being implemented by the BLS, procedures for the MCPI have involved pricing specific input items rather than obtaining average prices for episodes of treatment. For example, x-rays, laboratory tests, and physicians' office visits have been priced rather than the average price of treatment of, say, a child's forearm fracture.[11] Hence the MCPI ignores potential input substitution and much quality change, and it does not take changes in outcomes into account.

Although the MCPI currently employs fixed weights for the higher levels of aggregation based on the Consumer Expenditure Survey, at the lowest level of aggregation (entry-level items) the set of goods and services sampled are completely rotated over a five-year time period, and thus at least 20 percent of the sampled items change each year.[12]

Once items have been sampled, they are weighted and aggregated using a modified Laspeyres-type price index with fixed weights. Speci-

---

8. For further discussion, see Armknecht and Ginsburg (1992), especially pp. 124–42, and Fixler (1996).

9. Taken from U.S. Senate Finance Committee (1996), p. 63, table 2. The 1982–84 fixed weights were updated to 1993–95 weights beginning in January 1998.

10. See Dranove, Shanley, and White (1991).

11. For further discussion, see Armknecht and Ginsburg (1992); Cardenas (1996); Daugherty (1964); Ford and Sturm (1988); and Ginsburg (1978).

12. For further discussion in the context of a CPI for pharmaceuticals, see Cleeton, Goepfrich, and Weisbrod (1992).

fically, if the number of items sampled does not change, a price index could be computed using the traditional Laspeyres formula,

$$(3\text{-}1) \qquad L_t = \sum_{i=1}^{n} w_{i0}\left[\frac{p_{it}}{p_{i0}}\right]; \qquad w_{i0} = \frac{p_{i0}q_{i0}}{\displaystyle\sum_{i=1}^{n} p_{i0}q_{i0}},$$

where p_{it} is the price of the ith item in time period t, p_{i0} is the base period price, q_{i0} are fixed base period quantities, and w_{i0} is the fixed base period weight. When, as is typically the case, the sampled items change (because items are dropped out of the sample or new items are introduced from sample rotation or both), the BLS employs a modified and chained Laspeyres price index formula,

$$(3\text{-}2) \qquad L_t' = \sum_{i=1}^{n_{t-1}} w_{i,t-1}\left[\frac{p_{it}}{p_{i,t-1}}\right]\cdot L_{t-1}', \qquad w_{i,t-1} = \frac{p_{ib}q_{ib}}{\displaystyle\sum_{i=1}^{n_{t-1}} p_{i0}q_{i0}},$$

where the base period b could be that for time period 0, that for time period $t-1$, or some other time period.

For our purposes, it is sufficient to note that the BLS does not publish price indexes for the treatment of depression, although it does publish MCPIs for a physicians' services aggregate (that includes psychiatrists but does not identify their price series separately) and for an aggregate of prescription pharmaceutical drugs (but not for antidepressants as a separate category).

The BLS's PPI reflects average changes in selling prices received by domestic producers for their output.[13] Currently no aggregate medical care PPI is computed or published by the BLS. PPIs for various medical commodities (for example, pharmaceuticals, ophthalmic goods, medical instruments) have been published for quite some time as PPIs for distinct manufacturing industries. PPIs for health services industries are quite new; the BLS's hospital PPI was initiated in December 1992, a physicians' services PPI in December 1993, and a composite health services PPI in December 1994. Among the industries within the health services PPI, the

13. For further discussion of the PPI, see Catron and Murphy (1996); and Early and Sinclair (1983); see Heffler and others (1996).

BLS publishes monthly price data for six aggregates, including offices and clinics of doctors of medicine (with twelve separate components, including psychiatry), skilled and intermediate care facilities, general medical and surgical hospitals (a large category, with a separate index for mental diseases and disorders, among others), psychiatric hospitals, specialty hospitals except psychiatric, and medical laboratories.

The PPI includes revenues from Medicare, Medicaid, and other private sources (such as third-party insurance and direct patient cash payments). For hospitals, the unit of output is the services performed during a single hospital visit. Based on ICD-9 (International Classification of Diseases, 9th revision) and DRG (diagnostic related group) data from, among others, the Health Care Financing Administration randomly selected itemized patient bills are chosen to form a sample frame, and then the components of these itemized bills are repriced monthly. For physicians' services, the unit of output is represented by the patient's bill covering the services provided by a physician during a single patient-physician encounter. Note that while the PPI sample frame is based on prices from a selected actual treatment bundle, the PPI assumes use of identical inputs over time and thus does not allow for changes in the components of the treatment bundle, for example, substitution of prescription drugs for psychotherapy in the treatment of depression. Moreover, the PPI attempts to obtain net transaction prices that may vary by payer rather than list prices, but as of 1995, 43.4 percent of its sampled inpatient price quotes and 64.6 percent of its outpatient price quotes were based on list prices.[14]

Definition and Measurement of the Price for the Treatment of Depression

We now provide some background information on the nature of the illness known as major depression, its diagnosis, various forms of treatment for acute-phase major depression, and research findings on comparisons of treatment efficacy for specific forms of major depression. We then define alternative treatment bundles.

Major Depression

Depression is commonly characterized by melancholy, diminished interest and pleasure in all or most activities, and feelings of worthless-

---

14. Catron and Murphy (1996), table 4 and appendix 2.

ness. The clinical definition of major depression provides a very specific set of clinical criteria that must be met in order for a patient's condition to be considered an episode of major depression. Specifically, the *Diagnostic and Statistical Manual of Mental Disorders* of the American Psychiatric Association, fourth edition (DSM-IV), defines major depression as: "The presence of one of the first two symptoms, as well as at least five of nine total symptoms. The symptoms must be present most of the day almost every day, for at least two weeks. The symptoms include: 1. depressed mood most of the day nearly every day; 2. markedly diminished interest or pleasure in almost all activities most of the day; 3. significant weight loss/gain; 4. insomnia/hypersomnia; 5. psychomotor agitation/retardation; 6. feelings of worthlessness (guilt); 7. fatigue; 8. impaired concentration (indecisiveness); and 9. recurrent thoughts of death or suicide."[15]

There are two dimensions of depression with respect to persistence: single episode and recurrent major depression. A single episode is self-explanatory. Recurrent depression is defined by two or more major depressive episodes each separated by at least eight weeks of return to usual functioning.[16] Episodes of depression are also classified according to severity: mild, moderate, or severe. Mild depression typically involves the minimum number of symptoms required to meet clinical criteria and minor functional impairment. Moderately severe episodes are characterized by an excess in symptoms above the minimum to meet clinical criteria and by greater degrees of functional impairment. Severe major depression involves a number of excess symptoms above the minimum and significant degrees of functional impairment, including the inability to work or conduct usual activities.

Epidemiological studies indicate that in the early 1990s, 10.3 percent of the U.S. population met the criteria for major depression at some time during a twelve-month period.[17] The vast majority of individuals who experience an episode of major depression return to their original level of functioning. However, 20–35 percent experience persistent symptoms; these cases are commonly referred to as chronic depression. Furthermore, approximately 50 percent of all people having depressive episodes can be expected to have a recurrence.[18] Once an individual has a second episode, recurrence is 70 percent likely.

15. American Psychiatric Association (1994), p. 161.
16. See American Psychiatric Association (1993).
17. Kessler and others (1994), p. 12.
18. American Psychiatric Association (1993).

Alternative Treatments

In this research we focus on treatment for the acute phase of care. Research on the continuation phase of treatment is less developed, and definitive protocols have not been as widely adopted in many clinical settings. Treatments for major depression have advanced rapidly during the past twenty years. In the area of psychotherapy a variety of new techniques has expanded treatment options well beyond psychodynamic or psychoanalytic approaches. Interpersonal therapy, behavior therapy, family therapy, and cognitive behavior therapy are each relatively new. Evidence from controlled clinical trials suggests that when applied as the single mode of treatment for less severe forms of acute major depression, each of these therapies reduces depressive symptoms. Moreover, relative to antidepressive medication as the sole treatment, each has generally been shown to perform at comparable levels of efficacy and to have similar outcomes.[19]

Extraordinary advances have been achieved in the area of antidepressant medication. Over the 1991–95 time period covered by our claims data, there are three general classes of antidepressant medication: (1) cyclic antidepressants, which include the widely used tricyclic antidepressants (TCAs) and a number of lesser-known drugs such as trazodone; (2) selective serotonin reuptake inhibitors (SSRIs), which include brand-name drugs such as Prozac, Zoloft, Paxil, and Luvox; and (3) monoamine oxidase (MAO) inhibitors which, due to side effects and dangerous interactions, are generally used only for cases that are resistant to other forms of treatment. The newer SSRIs offer some distinct advantages over older TCAs. SSRIs are associated with lower risk of overdose as well as fewer and lower levels of a number of side effects. Key side effects associated with TCAs include drowsiness, dry mouth, impaired ability to concentrate, seizures, and weight gain.[20] SSRIs have been associated with side effects related to sexual dysfunction and anxiety. The advantages of SSRIs come at a significantly higher pecuniary cost than most TCAs.

Psychotherapeutic interventions have frequently been combined with antidepressant medication as a strategy for treating major depression. The specific interventions that have been most intensively studied are the use of TCAs in combination with either interpersonal therapy, behavior

---

19. See Beach, Sandeen, and O'Leary (1990); Beck and others (1979); Elkin and others (1989); Frank and others (1990); and Kupfer and others (1992).

20. It should be noted that there is considerable variation in side effects among the TCAs. See Berndt, Cockburn, and Griliches (1996), pp. 142–43, table 1, for details.

therapy, or a general unspecified form of short-term psychotherapy. No studies have been reported in the literature at this time that systematically assess the combination of SSRIs and psychotherapy. It is generally presumed that such combinations will be at least as efficacious as the combination of TCAs and psychotherapy.

Electroconvulsive therapy can be quite effective but is typically limited to rather special circumstances where the depression is severe and complicated by a number of other psychiatric symptoms, including psychosis, catatonic stupor, or high risk of suicide. In the analysis of treatment bundles presented here we focus on outpatient treatments for major depression, which constitute the vast majority of treatment episodes (75–80 percent). There are several reasons for this choice. First, inpatient claims do not contain information on the drugs prescribed for treatment; thus our characterization of inpatient care would be incomplete. A second reason for focusing on outpatient care is that it is more difficult to use administrative data to make judgments about the appropriate use of inpatient hospital services for treating depression. Finally, because there was considerable evidence of overuse of hospital services in the aggregate during the late 1980s and early 1990s, the inclusion of hospital services in a base year such as 1991 would create a downward bias in price changes as general reductions in the use of psychiatric hospitals occurred. We therefore focus on the use of various drugs alone, several forms of psychotherapy alone, and several drug-psychotherapy combination treatments; we do not incorporate electroconvulsive therapy or the MAO inhibitors.

We now turn to a brief discussion on research results concerning the efficacy of alternative treatments for depression of varying severity. A typical treated population consists of patients with varying levels of severity, and for given levels of severity, alternative treatments are provided. We develop a set of treatment "bundles" that groups therapies in "therapeutically similar groups" for treatment of a specific form of major depression. Our goal here is to identify treatment bundles that result in similar expected mental health outcomes. Our implicit assumption is that obtaining similar outcomes from alternative treatments begins to approximate similar utility levels.[21]

We divide levels of depression into two classes: severe and less severe (hereafter, mild). In order to classify therapies into therapeutically simi-

---

21. We recognize that this is only an approximation, especially for depression, where the constellation of side effects across treatments can differ significantly. Further indications of differences in preferences are reflected in the differential compliance with SSRI and other drug treatments. See Crown and others (1996).

lar treatment bundles, we have reviewed approximately thirty major clinical trials and meta-analyses from the clinical literature dealing with acute-phase treatment.[22] This literature points to several key conclusions:

First, psychotherapies of all kinds have been shown to result in superior outcomes compared to no treatment. When compared among themselves, the different forms of psychotherapy appear to have no significant differences in outcomes. The Agency for Health Care Policy and Research (AHCPR) provides a summary and interpretation of the evidence on this point.[23]

Second, for less severe forms of depression, psychotherapies alone, TCAs with medical management, TCAs alone, and SSRIs alone appear to produce comparable outcomes. All of the therapies tested produced significantly better outcomes than placebo treatments. Versions of these results have been reported in numerous large treatment trials and by meta-analyses of smaller clinical trials. Combination treatments with these as components also generate equivalent levels of efficacy for less severe forms of depression.

Third, for more severe forms of depression, the bulk of the evidence suggests that TCAs alone, SSRIs alone, and combinations of drugs and psychotherapy have comparable levels of efficacy, and each results in superior outcomes compared to psychotherapy alone. Recently some evidence has emerged showing some extra improvement from the combination treatments relative to medication alone.[24] We believe it is premature to conclude that combination treatments offer significantly higher levels of efficacy than do drugs alone (or with medical management, as is typically the case).

Based on these observations from the literature, we view all the major treatment technologies as offering comparable expected outcomes for the average care of less severe acute-phase depression. For severe depression we view TCAs and SSRIs alone as comparable to each other and to combinations of TCAs and SSRIs with psychotherapy.

Treatment Bundles for Depression

To determine prices of treatment bundles for depression we use a data set consisting of insurance claims for four large self-insured employers that offered twenty-five health plans to 428,168 enrollees and their de-

---

22. See Busch, Frank, and Berndt (1996).
23. See Depression Guideline Panel (1993); also see Elkin and others (1989).
24. See American Psychiatric Association (1993).

pendents. The data were obtained from MEDSTAT Inc. and contain information for the years 1991 through 1995. Information on drug claims, inpatient hospital treatment, outpatient visits, diagnoses, procedures, and the demographic characteristics of all employees are reported. The health insurance benefits offered to enrollees are generally quite generous relative to the general market for private health insurance in the United States. The mental health benefits are especially generous relative to typical private insurance (as will become evident in the discussion about cost sharing below). During the five years observed there were important changes in the terms of mental health coverage. While the majority of plans represent so-called managed indemnity plans (90–94 percent), the management of mental health care changed for a substantial number of enrollees between 1991 and 1995. Beginning on January 1, 1994, about 33 percent of the enrollees' mental health coverage was "carved out" to a specialty managed care company. In January 1995 an additional 16 percent of enrollees had their mental health benefits carved out.[25] These changes are expected to affect both the input prices and quantities of specific services delivered (for example, visits). Managed care arrangements have also been shown to affect the general clinical strategies used in treating depression. Recent analyses by Berndt, Frank, and McGuire and by Wells and others show clear differences in treatment patterns between managed care plans and indemnity insurance, with managed arrangements being associated with a higher likelihood of using prescription drug treatments.[26]

In developing our treatment bundles we focus on the outpatient claims and the prescription drug files. By focusing on outpatient treatment we reduce the number of observed severe cases of depression. Each outpatient and drug claim can accommodate two ICD-9 diagnostic codes. The point of departure was to identify cases of major depression. ICD-9 codes 296.2 (major depressive disorder—single episode) and 296.3 (major depressive disorder—recurrent episode) were used to define depression.[27] Using the diagnostic information and dates contained in the claims, we construct episodes of treatment. In the case of prescription drugs, we

25. Specialty carve-out arrangements occur when a portion of the health risk is managed separately from the rest of health care. For another discussion of these arrangements, see Frank, McGuire, and Newhouse (1995).

26. Berndt, Frank, and McGuire (1997); Wells and others (1996).

27. We exclude the remaining 296 ICD-9 diagnoses as well as some other broad depression-related conditions, such as neurotic depression.

consider the number of days of treatment provided by the prescription as the time period for which an individual received care. We follow previous research in identifying episodes of treatment as ending when no treatment is received for a period of time.[28] Specifically, the Practice Guidelines for Major Depressive Disorder in Adults of the American Psychiatric Association (APA) define an episode of depression as new if a diagnosis is preceded by a period of eight weeks of not meeting clinical criteria for depression.[29] Since we do not directly observe symptoms in claims data, we cannot make our claims-based definition of an episode of care correspond directly to an episode of illness.[30]

In defining our episodes of care we use an eight-week period without treatment to separate treatment episodes.[31] Applying these criteria, we defined 20,603 episodes of care for the five years, 1991–95. Censoring of episodes occurred at both the beginning of 1991 and at the end of 1995. Because we cannot fully observe the treatment received for the censored cases, we confine our attention to the 13,324 uncensored episodes in which we observe at least eight weeks without treatment at both the beginning and end of the episode. In order to limit the samples to less severe forms of major depression, we eliminated individuals with episodes involving inpatient hospital treatment for any mental illness at any time during the five years. This reduced the number of episodes to 10,368. Using information on treatment procedures (for example, type of visit) described by the CPT codes, we describe the composition of outpatient treatment that occurred within a treatment episode.

Drug treatment is based on the national drug codes reported on the claim. The national drug code classification of antidepressant medications revealed use of seven TCAs, three SSRIs, three MAO inhibitors, four anxiolytics, and four heterocyclics for treatment of depression.[32] The data show that 45 percent of the drug claims involved SSRIs, 22 percent TCAs, 19 percent anxiolytics, and 10 percent heterocyclics. These figures

28. Kessler (1980).

29. American Psychiatric Association (1993).

30. For a useful discussion of defining episodes of care, see Keeler and others (1986); and Wingert and others (1995).

31. As implied above, we count days without treatment only after the number of days of supply in a drug prescription has been exhausted, thereby assuming full compliance with the daily recommended dosage.

32. The anxiolytics are not indicated by the Federal Drug Administration for treatment of depression but could be prescribed for comorbid conditions associated with depression and/or as responses to side effects from antidepressants.

are consistent with IMS aggregate national sales data for antidepressant medication reported by Berndt, Cockburn, and Griliches.[33]

For this initial analysis we only consider "pure" treatments. That is, we only consider episodes of care that correspond directly to treatments tested in the clinical trials literature. In this way we can directly link the "price" of an episode of a well-defined treatment to the price of other therapeutically similar treatments.

We identify nine major classes of treatment that have been proven effective in the treatment of depression: (1) psychotherapy alone, 6–15 visits; (2) short-term TCA treatment alone or with medical management, 30–180 days; (3) short-term SSRI treatment alone or with medical management, 30–180 days; (4) short-term TCA treatment of 30–180 days with some psychotherapy; (5) short-term SSRI treatment (30–180 days) with some psychotherapy. The four remaining treatments are identical to the last four above, except for the provision of anxiolytic medication.

In order to improve the precision of the estimated mean "prices" of treatment bundles, we aggregate several closely related bundles (for example, short-term SSRI treatment with an anxiolytic drug and short-term SSRI treatment alone). The result was five treatment bundles used in the analyses reported here. We also examine a set of fourteen treatment bundles that relax the criteria for inclusion that defined the nine pure treatments discussed above. This larger set of treatments nearly accords with guideline standards and accounts for 20–40 percent of episodes.

As previously mentioned, when claims data were converted to uncensored episodes of major depression, 10,368 episodes of depression were identified. Based on the definitions noted above, the number of episodes treated with each of the nine pure protocol treatments was calculated. It is notable that of the 10,368 episodes identified, a substantial share of treatments (75–80 percent) do not resemble standard protocol treatments. For example, 1,818 episodes (47 percent of the 3,900) treated with psychotherapy alone consisted of a single visit. In addition, 1,672, or 16 percent of all episodes, received neither psychotherapy nor an antidepressant drug. As a result, the number of episodes receiving guideline standards of care was relatively small (20–25 percent).

The interpretation of the observed patterns of care is complex. For instance, in the case of single-visit episodes, those visits may have taken place for the purposes of "ruling out" major depression as the relevant

---

33. Berndt, Cockburn, and Griliches (1996).

condition to be treated in favor of a somatic condition or another mental disorder. In this case, the visit should not be viewed as "inappropriate treatment" but as an appropriate assessment. Indeed, the depression guidelines published by AHCPR state: "Effective treatment rests on accurate diagnosis. The practitioner must first determine whether the patient has a clinical depression or is simply suffering normal sadness or distress. . . . For patients who have very mild cases of major depression or whose diagnosis is unclear and who are not in immediate danger or are not suffering significant functional impairment, the practitioner may want to schedule one or two additional weekly evaluation visits to determine whether symptoms will abate without formal treatment."[34]

For this reason, distinguishing treatment and assessment is very difficult with claims data. The implication is that we are somewhat uncertain as to whether 20–40 percent of care lies on the production frontier or whether 30–45 percent of treatments are close to the frontier. With this as a caveat, we now examine the various treatment bundles in greater detail.

PSYCHOTHERAPY. Of the 10,368 episodes, 3,900 (38 percent) were treated with psychotherapy alone. No distinction was made in the claims data between different types of psychotherapy. Considering the 2,802 treatments involving fifty-minute psychotherapy sessions, we find that 2,094 (75 percent) received five or fewer visits and 1,140 (41 percent) only a single visit.

A total of 1,098 episodes were treated with psychotherapy sessions of twenty minutes' duration without antidepressant medication (eight of those treatments included anxiolytic medication). Of those, 863 episodes (78 percent) were treated with just a single short visit, and 198 episodes (18 percent) were treated with between two and five short sessions. An additional twenty-six episodes (2 percent) were treated with some form of group therapy, with only half of those treatments involving more than three visits.

While clinical trials data indicate that individuals typically show partial response to psychotherapy by six weeks of treatment (with weekly sessions) and remission in twelve weeks, published guidelines for the treatment of the acute phase of depression do not indicate any demonstrated effectiveness for fewer than six visits. The benefits of short psychotherapy visits, in the absence of antidepressant medication, have not been studied

34. Depression Guideline Panel (1993), p. 36.

and therefore cannot be considered either effective or ineffective treatment. Although clinical trials and published treatment guidelines indicate psychotherapeutic treatment is an effective treatment, in our data of the 2,802 episodes given this treatment, only 708 episodes (25 percent) can be considered to have completed a psychotherapy regimen that is consistent with guideline treatments.[35]

ANTIDEPRESSANT MEDICATION. Claims data do not include information on how many days medication was actually taken, so we use as a proxy the number of days of treatment for which a prescription was filled. Our data also do not provide adequate information on the dose of medication; moreover, the definition of an adequate dose varies by individual. For these two reasons, our estimates of individuals receiving clinically proven effective treatment may be conservative.

Of the 10,368 episodes considered, 224 were treated with TCA either alone (186) or in combination with anxiolytic medication (38). Of these 224 episodes, 65 (29 percent) were treated with less than thirty days of medication and 45 with ten or fewer days. Generally, the clinical literature (and the APA guidelines) indicate that while patients may show some improvement to antidepressant medication by the end of the first week, full response to acute-phase depression may take four to six weeks.

An additional 765 episodes were treated with SSRIs either alone (635) or in combination with anxiolytic medication (130). Of these episodes, 105 (17 percent) were treated with fewer than thirty days of medication. Because individuals have different reactions to drugs, some individuals are appropriately treated with one class of antidepressants and then switched to another class. In our sample 470 episodes were treated with both TCAs and SSRIs.

USE OF OTHER PRESCRIPTION DRUGS. Several episodes were treated with drugs other than SSRIs and TCAs. In our sample 10 episodes were treated with MAO inhibitors, and 64 were treated with heterocyclics. An additional 131 episodes were treated with anti-anxiety medication alone, a protocol that has not been approved by the FDA for the treatment of depression. The use of alprazolam may be appropriate if other medication is contraindicated, but there is no evidence for the efficacious use of other anxiolytic medications.[36]

---

35. For a related discussion, see Katon and others (1992).
36. See Wells and others (1994, 1996) for further discussion.

COMBINATION TREATMENTS. The share of episodes treated with a combination treatment involving both psychotherapy and an antidepressant grew over the time period considered, from 34 percent in 1991 to 48 percent in 1994. Overall, 404 treatments consisted of both some TCA and some psychotherapy, and 1,491 included both SSRI and some psychotherapy. A large share of the episodes treated with combination treatments had three or fewer psychotherapy visits (48 percent). An additional 363 episodes were treated with some TCA, some SSRI, and some psychotherapy.

COMPARISON WITH RESULTS FROM OTHER STUDIES. The patterns of care observed in this data set raise issues related to the likely effectiveness of treatment in the presence of efficacious treatment technologies. One potential criticism of the patterns of treatment bundle data presented above is that they are based on claims data. Claims data are useful in that the retrospective medical treatment of many individuals can be analyzed efficiently and at minimal expense. In addition, such observational data indicate the "real world" practice of medicine. Claims data are also used for quality assessment by organizations constructing "report cards" on health care organizations. Yet claims data have been fairly criticized for several reasons. The accuracy of diagnoses and recorded data are sometimes questioned and omissions in records are common. For example, depression has been shown to be underdiagnosed by primary care physicians and overdiagnosed by psychiatric clinicians.[37]

Other studies have found less dramatic but corresponding treatment patterns for depression. The medical outcomes study consists of 635 individuals diagnosed with depression or with current depressive symptoms for whom data were collected by self-administered questionnaires, patient diaries, phone interviews, and health exams. The study found that only 23 percent of depressed patients had used an antidepressant medication in the prior month or used it daily for a month or more in the prior six months. Of those patients using an antidepressant medication, 39 percent used an inappropriately low dose.[38]

The medical outcomes study did not report number of psychotherapy visits. Instead, it reported "counseling," which it defined as three or more minutes of counseling during the screening interview. This makes comparison with published standards on care difficult. Although 90 percent

37. See Schulberg and others (1985).
38. Wells and others (1994).

of patients of mental health specialists were counseled, among general medical practitioners where most study participants were treated, only 20 percent of managed care and 40 percent of fee-for-service patients were counseled.

Another study of eighty-eight outpatients enrolled in the National Institute of Mental Health Clinical Research Collaborative Program on the Psychobiology of Depression: Clinical Study found that only 19 percent of patients received an adequate dose and duration of antidepressant medication, and 24 percent received some anti-anxiety medication. Regarding psychotherapy visits, 44 percent were seen for at least one hour weekly.[39] Although these two studies have somewhat higher rates of treatments that have been shown to be efficacious than we observe in our claims data, these patients and their physicians knew they were participating in research studies, and since patients had sought care, one would expect to observe higher rates of utilization. Thus the low levels of efficacious treatments found in the medical outcomes study and National Institute of Mental Health studies, while surprising, are consistent with the treatment patterns found in the claims data we observe here.

For our purposes of constructing price indexes for the treatment of depression, we must make a decision as to whether to utilize the data suggesting treatment not consistent with FDA approvals and AHCPR guidelines. Since the interpretation of such treatments is problematic, we confine our attention to episodes of treatment defined as being consistent with AHCPR guidelines. Additional research on guideline-incompatible care is currently under way.

Prices of Treatment Bundles

In table 3-1 we report the average supply (PPI) and demand (CPI) "prices" of each of the five aggregated treatment bundles in 1991 and 1995. The PPI in table 3-1 measures the supply price, which includes both the payment made by the health plan and the patient's out-of-pocket payments to the provider. The CPI reports the out-of-pocket payments or consumer demand price components for the same bundles, that is, the copayments or deductible contribution made by the patient-consumer.

Table 3-1 reveals rather dramatic differences in the supply "price" of treatment bundles for depression. This is even the case for therapeutically similar bundles. For example, short-term psychotherapy alone (5–15 vis-

---

39. Keeler and others (1986).

Table 3-1. *Average Costs of Treatment, 1991*

Short-term treatment	Number of psychotherapy visits	Drug regimen (days)	N	Anxiolytics allowed?	PPI *(dollars)*[a]	CPI *(dollars)*[a]
Psychotherapy	5–15	0	78 (197)	no	924 (646)	151 (95)
Tricyclic antidepressants	0	30–180	18 (8)	yes	267 (117)	25 (39)
Selective serotonin reuptake inhibitors	0	30–180	33 (66)	yes	254 (214)	11 (21)
Psychotherapy and tricyclic antidepressants	1–15	30–180	25 (13)	yes	791 (391)	124 (59)
Psychotherapy and selective serotonin reuptake inhibitors	1–15	30–180	41 (128)	yes	762 (582)	103 (90)

Source: Authors' calculations.
a. 1995 values in parentheses.

its) has an estimated price of about $924 during the 1991 base year. In contrast, short-term TCA treatment alone (30–180 days) is priced at about $267 if assessment and medical management costs are included, and SSRI alone (30–180 days) is slightly lower at $254 per episode. Note that all three of these treatments have similar levels of efficacy for treatment of acute-phase less severe depression, even though the total costs per episode of treatment range by a factor of almost four, from $924 to $254.

Table 3-1 also shows even greater relative variation in the consumer demand price across treatments. For example, the demand price for the psychotherapy alone bundle is $151, whereas TCA and SSRI treatments alone are about $25 and $11. The implied patient copayment-deductible percentage contributions for short-term psychotherapy alone, TCA alone, and SSRI alone are 16 percent, 9 percent, and 4 percent, respectively. From the patient's vantage, therefore, the required out-of-pocket-payments percentage is highest for psychotherapy alone and lowest for SSRI alone.

The estimated prices for the combined treatments are generally based on a smaller number of cases and should therefore be viewed as less reliable. The most common form of mixed treatment is a combination of at least one psychotherapy visit along with a 30–180 day protocol level of treatment with an SSRI. In that case the supply price is $762 and the demand price $103 (14 percent of supply price). Psychotherapy with TCA is estimated to have a supply price of $791 and a demand price of $124 (16 percent of supply price). Thus relative supply prices are quite comparable largely due to the extra monitoring associated with TCAs.

Table 3-1 reports the supply and demand prices for 1995 in parentheses in the final two columns of the table. Nominal supply prices for all five treatment bundles fell over the five years. In some cases the price decreases were substantial, such as the 30 percent fall in the price of psychotherapy alone. This was due primarily to a decrease in the price of psychotherapy visits as opposed to a reduction in the number of visits within the acceptable range. Specifically, the mean number of visits for episodes treated with psychotherapy alone fell from 8.05 visits in 1991 to 7.7 visits in 1995. While the fall in drug treatment supply prices appears to be largely due to a fall in quantity (duration of drug treatments in the SSRI-alone category fell from 90 to 69 days), this result is primarily an artifact of censoring and quantity remains essentially constant.

Construction of Price Indexes

We now outline the construction of PPIs and CPIs for the treatment of depression. Recall that based on information from the medical literature, we are able to collect different types of treatment into groups with basically similar expected efficacy. We began with the nine bundles of treatment that are similarly efficacious for the treatment of acute-phase mild depression. In order to increase the precision of the estimated mean bundle prices we aggregated the nine bundles into five. In this section we present price indexes for the five bundles. We have also constructed price indexes using the fourteen bundles based on the broader criteria for inclusion of observed treatments.

Price Indexes Examined

Alternative formulae for constructing price indexes correspond to differing assumptions on the extent of ex ante substitutability among the treatment bundles. Denote the quantity of bundle i in year t as B_{it}, and its supply price as P_{it}; set the base period (say, 1991) quantities and prices at B_{i0} and P_{i0}.

One possible approach is to assume that in spite of their therapeutic similarity, the treatment bundles are completely nonsubstitutable, with idiosyncratic patients expected to respond to only one form of treatment. The Laspeyres fixed base-period quantity weight formula in equation (3-1) is implied by this zero substitutability assumption and results in the following price index formula:

$$(3\text{-}3) \qquad\qquad I_t^L = \frac{\sum\limits_{i=1}^{5} p_{it} B_{i0}}{\sum\limits_{i=1}^{5} p_{i0} B_{i0}}.$$

A fixed-weight Paasche index is computed in an analogous manner, but the fixed quantity weights are those of the final time period.

An alternative extreme assumption is that consumers cannot differentiate at all among the alternative treatments. One way of implementing this is simply to compare the price over all episodes treated in year t to the average price over all treated episodes in the base period:

$$(3\text{-}4) \qquad\qquad I_t^P = \frac{\sum\limits_{i=1}^{5} \dfrac{p_{it} B_{i0}}{B_t}}{\sum\limits_{i=1}^{5} \dfrac{p_{i0} B_{i0}}{B_0}},$$

where $B_0 = \sum\limits_{i=1}^{5} B_{i0}$ and B_t is analogous. We call this a "perfect substitutability" price index.

Two other alternatives involve less extreme assumptions. If one assumes that the elasticity of substitution between treatment bundles is unity, then one can construct the Cobb-Douglas index as

$$(3\text{-}5) \qquad\qquad I_t^C = \frac{\prod\limits_{i=1}^{5} P_{it}^{w_i}}{\prod\limits_{i=1}^{5} P_{i0}^{w_i}},$$

which in logarithmic form is written as

(3-6) $$\ln I_t^C = \sum_{i=1}^{5} w_i \ln\left(\frac{P_{it}}{P_{i0}}\right),$$

where the w_i are fixed expenditure share weights, computed as, say, the mean expenditure shares for each of the five bundles over the 1991–95 time period.

Finally, as Diewert has shown, one can compute a Tornqvist discrete approximation to the continuous Divisia index that makes no *a priori* assumption about the elasticity of substitution among the five treatment bundles.[40] It is worth noting, incidentally, that use of the discrete Divisia index is consistent with the recommendations of the CPI Commission, whereas use of the other index numbers is not. Letting I_t^T denote the value of the Tornqvist discrete approximation to the Divisia price index, calculate this index as

(3-7) $$\ln\left(\frac{I_t^T}{I_{t-1}^T}\right) = \sum_{i=1}^{5} \overline{w}_{it} \ln\left(\frac{P_{it}}{P_{i,t-1}}\right),$$

where the time varying mean expenditure shares $\overline{w}_{it} \equiv \dfrac{(w_{it} + w_{i,t-1})}{2}$, and

(3-8) $$w_{it} \equiv \frac{P_{it} B_{it}}{\sum_{i=1}^{5} P_{it} B_{it}}.$$

The Laspeyres and Paasche price indexes can involve either fixed or sequentially updated or chained quantity weights. In the fixed-weight Laspeyres we employ 1991 weights, whereas in the fixed-weight Paasche we employ 1995 weights. Laspeyres and Paasche indexes with chained weights are also computed. A common finding from other price index research is that the chained Tornqvist index falls in between the chained Laspeyres and Paasche indexes.[41]

To this point we have not specified precisely what prices and quantities B_{it} one would employ in these index number calculations. In the case of the Laspeyres index of equation (3-4), we use mean treatment bundle

40. Diewert (1976).
41. Ibid.

"prices" for each of the five aggregate bundles (built up from the nine efficacious bundles identified in the data). We follow the same approach for the other indexes as well. Note also that while the above discussion has focused on the construction of a PPI (supply price), the construction of a CPI (demand price) proceeds in an analogous manner.

Results of Price Indexes 1991–95

Tables 3-2 and 3-3 report the results of constructing the PPI and CPI versions of the price indexes discussed above, as well as of using the five aggregate treatment bundles. The results for Laspeyres, Paasche, Perfect Substitutes, Cobb-Douglas, and Tornqvist indexes reported in table 3-2 offer a consistent view of price movements for acute-phase treatment of major depression. Specifically, the fixed-weight Laspeyres, Paasche, and Cobb-Douglas indexes all indicate supply "price" reductions of about 30 percent over the 1991–95 period. The fixed-weight Laspeyres index shows the largest fall, to an index value of 68.4 compared to values of 70.6 for both the fixed-weight Paasche and the chained Laspeyres. The perfect substitutes index value for the PPI fell to 77.1 by 1995. The chained and fixed-weight Paasche indexes, as well as the chained Tornqvist, show similar price declines of about 28 percent; the 1995 indexes are 71.8, 71.9, and 71.2, respectively (1991 = 100).

Thus although all price indexes reveal a decline in the supply price of treating acute-phase depression in a manner consistent with AHCPR guidelines, the extent of the decline varies modestly with the choice of weights and substitution assumptions. The fact that we observe this sensitivity to choice of weights in turn implies that weights must have changed during the 1991–95 time period.

Among the changes occurring in the market for mental health services, we expect to observe substitution across treatment bundles over time, from more psychotherapy-intensive and expensive care to greater utilization of lower-cost drug and less psychotherapy-intensive care. Figure 3-1 reflects the changes in the quantity weights for the five treatment bundles. This figure reveals several important trends that have been noted more generally in the treatment of depression. It should be pointed out that 1995 represents a departure from the trend in the four previous years.[42] One important trend is the shift toward treatments that make use

---

42. During the 1991–94 period the number of treatments rose steadily from 195 cases to 564. The number of cases fell in 1995 to 412. This is an artifact of censoring. The 1995 results are puzzling and possibly anomalous.

Table 3-2. *Producer Price Index (PPI) for Five Aggregate Treatment Bundles*

Percent

	1991	1992	1993	1994	1995
Research indexes, depression					
Laspeyres, fixed-weight	100	98.4	86.7	79.2	68.4
Chained	100	98.4	86.1	81.9	70.6
Paasche, fixed-weight	100	98.3	88.9	82.1	71.9
Chained	100	99.3	84.9	82.0	71.8
Perfect substitutes	100	99.3	81.5	78.2	77.1
Cobb-Douglas	100	99.7	87.4	82.2	70.6
Tornqvist-chained	100	98.9	85.6	81.9	71.2
Comparison indexes, PPI					
Health services				100	102.4
Psychotherapeutics	400	430.7	453.5	464.7	481.7
	(100)	(107.6)	(113.4)	(116.2)	(120.4)
Inpatient treatment	n.a.	100	102.4	106.0	109.9

Source: Authors' calculations.

n.a. Not available.

a. Indexes normalized to 1991 or 1992 base in parentheses.

Table 3-3. *Consumer Price Index (CPI) for Five Aggregate Treatment Bundles*

Percent

	1991	1992	1993	1994	1995
Research indexes, depression					
Laspeyres, fixed-weight	100	91.3	83.7	79.6	70.2
Chained	100	91.3	84.0	81.8	77.7
Paasche, fixed-weight	100	87.6	84.5	80.9	71.9
Chained	100	90.9	83.7	83.0	73.8
Perfect substitutes	100	89.5	74.2	72.1	77.7
Cobb-Douglas	100	89.5	74.2	72.1	77.8
Tornqvist-chained	100	91.2	83.8	82.3	75.7
Comparison indexes					
Medical care services[a]	177.1	190.5	202.9	213.4	224.2
	(100)	(107.5)	(114.6)	(120.5)	(126.6)
Prescription drugs[a]	197.7	214.7	223.0	230.6	235.0
	(100)	(107.5)	(111.7)	(115.5)	(117.7)

Source: Authors' calculations.

a. Indexes normalized to 1991 base in parentheses.

Figure 3-1. *Quantity Shares of Short-Term Treatment Bundles*

Percent

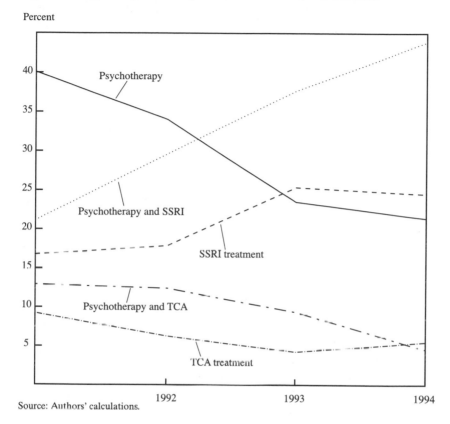

Source: Authors' calculations.

of SSRI drugs as inputs. This is evidenced by the increasing shares of mixed treatments using SSRI drugs and the general growth in use of SSRI drugs alone. The diminishing role of psychotherapy alone is shown in figure 3-1. For example, from 1991 to 1994 the psychotherapy-alone bundle quantity share fell from 40 to 21 percent, although it rebounded to 48 percent in 1995. Finally, treatments that use TCA drugs have declined as a share of all treatments for depression.

All of these price reductions are rather dramatic and contrast sharply to changes in the published medical PPIs. The final three rows of table 3-2 report the BLS's health services PPI, the psychotherapeutics category of the pharmaceutical PPI, and the inpatient general hospital PPI. All three of these indexes estimate price increases for mental health-related services. The psychotherapeutics index rises 20 percent during the 1991–95 period, while the inpatient treatment PPI increases about 10 percent between 1992 and 1995. The differential between the indexes for treatment of depression and, say, the psychotherapeutics PPI is on the order of 15 percent per year. One implication of these results is that analyses of expenditure data for mental health services are very likely confusing the price and volume components of care increases.

Table 3-3 reports the demand price for CPI results. As in the case of the PPI, the demand prices for acute-phase treatment of depression have moved downward during the 1991–95 period. The price reductions have ranged from 22 percent for the Cobb-Douglas and perfect substitution indexes to about 30 percent for the fixed-weight Laspeyres. As with the PPI, the sequentially updated chained Laspeyres and Paasche indexes reveal smaller price declines (about 22 percent and 26 percent, respectively) than their fixed-weight counterparts over the full 1991–95 time period. This result shows that fixed-weight indexes can be biased downward. The similarity between the PPI and CPI results in part reflects the stability in benefit design within the data set analyzed. Nevertheless some noteworthy differences are reflected in the Tornqvist index values. For the PPI the largest changes in price occur in 1993 and 1995. The CPI for depression shows large price reductions in 1992 and 1995, reflecting perhaps the differences in the level of out-of-pocket payments, stemming both from shifts of utilization across treatment bundles (as they are substituted) having different cost-sharing provisions (for example, psychotherapy versus drug treatments) as well as price falls within bundles (which are also reflected in the PPI).

In the bottom two rows of table 3-3 we report the BLS's medical care CPI (or the MCPI) and the CPI for prescription drugs. These serve to contrast the behavior of the price of treating acute-phase depression to the more common indexes that are applied to health and mental health services. As with its PPIs, the BLS CPI indexes that relate to mental health treatment have both increased substantially during the 1991–95 period. The MCPI increases nearly 27 percent while the prescription drug CPI increases by almost 18 percent. Again, the average annual differential between the depression indexes and the MCPI is on the order of 10–15 percent. Both the supply and demand price growth differentials from the BLS indexes are about three times larger than the 4.4 percent differential reported by Cutler, McClellan, and Newhouse (chapter 2) for heart attack treatment.

The analyses of mental health spending performed by the Health Care Financing Administration and actuaries in the analysis of legislative proposals typically rely on the MCPI and its components to project growth and composition of spending. An important implication of our results is that in such cases the composition of spending will result in a significant underestimate of growth in the quantity of effective care delivered and may also incorrectly project total spending into the future.

One concern with drawing inferences based on the indexes for treatment of acute-phase depression reported above is that by using relatively strict criteria for identifying effective care (guideline standards), we omit much of the care actually delivered that is not on the production frontier. We consider the implications of this point by relaxing the guideline criteria to include treatment episodes that were "near misses" of the guideline standards. This led us to define fourteen treatment bundles that accounted for between 20 and 40 percent (depending on the year) of all treatment episodes. The resulting recalculations of the indexes are quite similar both in terms of the qualitative finding of falling index values between 1991 and 1995 and the magnitude of the fall. Thus to the extent that we are able to expand criteria to increase substantially the share of total treatments on the frontier, we obtain price indexes with robust time trends from 1991 to 1995.[43]

Concluding Observations

The results reported here suggest that by constructing a price index for the treatment of a specific illness that uses the episode of care to define quantity, that attempts to incorporate outcome information in defining output, and that focuses on transactions prices for both suppliers and consumers, one obtains results that depart substantially from the MCPI and specific health care PPIs.[44] We began our investigation with the notion that this might well be the case as suggested, or conjectured, in earlier research.[45] Our results should be viewed as suggestive that the MCPI and PPIs may be particularly prone to distortion for medical treatments where (1) managed care has potentially large impacts on both input prices and the composition of treatment; and (2) there has been important technical change in treatment methods. This is certainly the case with the treatment of major depression. The substantial fall in prices for all index formulations is dramatic and points to potentially important

43. These results are available from the authors upon request.
44. Dranove, Shanley, and White (1991).
45. Scitovsky (1967); U.S. Senate Finance Committee (1996).

misinterpretations of spending data on mental health services over the past ten years. Specifically, our work points to the possibility that recent increases in spending are generated primarily by quantity increases in the volume of care delivered rather than input price increases. Nevertheless, our results represent only an initial examination of price indexes for the treatment of depression. A number of important issues need to be addressed before we can confidently arrive at conclusions about the movement of prices and quantities for the treatment of depression.

First, we have not accounted for quality differences across similarly effective treatment bundles. Characteristics of an individual's specific illness (for example, comorbid substance abuse, risk of suicide), the treatment (for example, likelihood and type of side effects), and the delivery system (for example, managed care) may affect the preferences of specific individuals (and their agents) for different treatment technologies. To account for this, hedonic prices could be estimated and corresponding quality-adjusted price indexes could be constructed. A second issue relates to the potential precision of estimated costs and shares for specific treatment bundles. While the data set used in the analysis consisted of more than 400,000 people, many of the specific treatment bundles in a given year contained only a small number of cases for estimating the "average price." Obtaining still larger databases is an important next step in the research program. A third issue concerns the characterization of the mental health production function used in the analysis above. We have defined treatments in terms of their adherence or proximity to patterns of care defined by practice guidelines. While this has the benefit of approximating an isoquant for the expected outcome of treatments for depression, it also implies a production function that has a "step function" shape. It is clear that there are treatments for particular classes of patients below and above the guideline levels of care where the expected outcome is positive and less, or greater, than that implied by the guideline treatments, thereby suggesting a more traditional shape for the production function. For this reason we believe that developing price indexes based on a broader characterization of the mental health production function is necessary to meet the normative assumptions underlying price indexes. We expect to find that the majority of treatments will lie on the more broadly defined production frontier. Nevertheless, our findings concerning the significant number of treatments involving a single therapy visit or inappropriate drug treatments does suggest that an important portion of the care received for treatment of depression may not be on the frontier.

The approach to price index calculation proposed here also raises practical problems if it is to be implemented by public statistical agencies. One potential problem concerning BLS implementation is that the retrospective claims data we have employed are typically not available in real time, but instead come with a lag of nine months to two years. Two possibilities come to mind that would still permit computation and publication of price indexes for episodes of treatment in a timely manner. First, the BLS could consider adding treatment questions to its survey form, questions that essentially replicate the information we have obtained from the retrospective claims that have enabled us to construct an average price-by-treatment bundle. Alternatively, the BLS could utilize the annual time series of supply price and demand prices of the final different treatment bundles and then regress these treatment bundle prices on the BLS's official PPI or CPI data on physician office visits, pharmaceuticals, and selected other variables;[46] parameters from such a regression equation could then be used along with existing CPI or PPI data to generate a preliminary predicted treatment bundle price. This preliminary predicted price could then be substituted into the preliminary price index, which could be calculated and published in a timely manner and then be revised as additional data became available.

Finally, a difficult issue we have not dealt with in this paper is how the CPI for treatment of episodes of a disease should deal with the fact that the typical insured patient has prepaid his or her health insurance, which then covers the nondeductible and noncopayment components of the supply price. Integrating the ex ante cost of insurance with the out-of-pocket-payments component to produce a readily interpretable MCPI is an important issue for future research.[47]

References

American Psychiatric Association. 1993. "Practice Guidelines for Major Depressive Disorder in Adults."American Journal of Psychiatry 150(4): 1–26.

———. 1994. *Diagnostic and Statistical Manual of Mental Disorders*. 4th ed. Washington, D.C.

Armknecht, Paul A., and Daniel H. Ginsburg. 1992. "Improvements in Measuring Price Changes in Consumer Services: Past, Present and Future." In *Output Measurement in the Service Sectors*, edited by Zvi Griliches, pp. 109–56. Conference on

46. We are currently investigating the possibility of employing a time series of data on incomes, wages, and hours of various psychotherapy providers, as collected by Psychotherapy Finances.

47. For discussions of this insurance issue, see Armknecht and Ginsburg (1992), especially pp. 124–42, Daugherty (1964); Fixler (1996); and Griliches (1992), especially pp. 11–13.

Research in Income and Wealth, Studies in Income and Wealth 56. University of Chicago Press for the National Bureau of Economic Research.

Beach, Steven R. H., Evelyn E. Sandeen, and K. Daniel O'Leary. 1990. *Depression in Marriage*. New York: Guilford Press.

Beck, A. T., and others. 1979. *Cognitive Therapy of Depression*. New York: Guilford Press.

Berndt, Ernst R., Iain Cockburn, and Zvi Griliches. 1996. "Pharmaceutical Innovations and Market Dynamics: Tracking Effects on Price Indexes for Antidepressant Drugs." *Brookings Papers on Economic Activity: Microeconomics 1996*, pp. 133–88.

Berndt, Ernst R., Richard G. Frank, and Thomas G. McGuire. 1997. "Alternative Insurance Arrangements and the Treatment of Depression: What Are the Facts?" *American Journal of Managed Care* 3(2): 243–50.

Busch, Susan H., Richard G. Frank, and Ernst R. Berndt. 1996. "Effectiveness, Efficacy and Price Indexes for Depression: A Review of the Literature." Harvard Medical School, Department of Health Care Policy.

Cardenas, Elaine. 1996. "The CPI for Hospital Services: Concepts and Procedures." *Monthly Labor Review* (July): 34–42.

Catron, Brian, and Bonnie Murphy. 1996. "Hospital Price Inflation: What Does the New PPI Tell Us?" *Monthly Labor Review* (July): 24–31.

Cleeton, David L., Valy T. Goepfrich, and Burton A. Weisbrod. 1992. "What Does the Consumer Price Index for Prescription Drugs Really Measure?" *Health Care Financing Review* 13(3): 45–51.

Crown, William E., and others. 1996. "Application of Sample Selection Models to Outcomes Research: The Case of Evaluating Effects of Antidepressant Therapy on Resource Utilization." MedStat Group, Cambridge, Mass.

Cutler, David M., and others. 1996. "Are Medical Prices Declining?" Working Paper 5750. Cambridge, Mass.: National Bureau of Economic Research.

Daugherty, J. C. 1964. "Health Insurance in the Revised CPI." *Monthly Labor Review* 87(11): 1299–300.

Depression Guideline Panel. 1993. *Depression in Primary Care*. Vol. 2. AHCPR publication 93-0551. Rockville, Md.: U.S. Department of Health and Human Services.

Diewert, W. Erwin. 1976. "Exact and Superlative Index Numbers." *Journal of Econometrics* 4(2): 115–46.

Dranove, David, Mark Shanley, and William D. White. 1991. "Does the Consumer Price Index Overstate Hospital Price Inflation?" *Medical Care* 29: 690–96.

Early, John F., and James H. Sinclair. 1983. "Quality Adjustment in the Producer Price Indexes." In *The U.S. National Income and Product Accounts: Selected Topics*, edited by Murray Foss, pp. 107–45. Conference on Research in Income and Wealth. University of Chicago Press for the National Bureau of Economic Research.

Elkin, Irene, and others. 1989. "National Institute of Mental Health Treatment of Depression Collaborative Research Program: General Effectiveness of Treatments." *Archives of General Psychiatry* 46: 971–82.

Fixler, Dennis. 1996. "The Treatment of the Price of Health Insurance in the CPI." U.S. Department of Labor, Bureau of Labor Statistics, Washington, D.C.

Ford, I. Kay, and P. Sturm. 1988. "CPI Revision Provides More Accuracy in the Medical Care Services Component." *Monthly Labor Review* 111(4): 17–26.

Frank, Ellen, and others. 1990. "Three-year Outcomes for Maintenance Therapies in Recurrent Depression." *Archives of General Psychiatry* 47: 1093–99.

Frank, R. G., T. G. McGuire, and J. P. Newhouse. 1995. "Risk Contracts in Managed Mental Health Care." *Health Affairs* 14(3): 50–64.

Getzen, Thomas E. 1992. "Medical Care Price Indexes: Theory, Construction and Empirical Analysis of the U.S. Series 1927-1990." In *Advances in Health Economics and Health Services Research*, edited by Richard M. Scheffler and Louis F. Rossiter, pp. 83–128. Vol. 13. Greenwich, Conn.: JAI Press.

Gilbert, M. 1961. "The Problem of Quality Change and Index Numbers." *Monthly Labor Review* 84(9): 992–97.

———. 1962. "Quality Change and Index Numbers: A Reply." *Monthly Labor Review* 85(5): 544–45.

Ginsburg, Daniel H. 1978. "Medical Care Services in the Consumer Price Index." *Monthly Labor Review* 101(8): 35–39.

Greenberg, Paul E., and others. 1993. "The Economic Burden of Depression in 1990." *Journal of Clinical Psychiatry* 54(11): 405–18.

Griliches, Zvi. 1962. "Quality Change and Index Numbers: A Critique." *Monthly Labor Review* 85(5): 532–44.

———. 1992. "Introduction." In *Output Measurement in the Service Sectors*, edited by Zvi Griliches, pp. 1–22. Conference on Research in Income and Wealth, Studies in Income and Wealth 56. University of Chicago Press for the National Bureau of Economic Research.

Heffler, Stephen K., and others. 1996. "Hospital, Employment, and Price Indicators for the Health Care Industry: Fourth Quarter 1995 and Annual Data for 1987–95." *Health Care Financing Review* 17(4): 217–56.

Katon, Wayne, and others. 1992. "Adequacy and Duration of Antidepressant Treatment in Primary Care." *Medical Care* 30: 67–76.

Keeler, Emmett B., and others. 1986. "The Demand for Episodes of Mental Health Services." RAND Report R-3432-NIMH, Santa Monica, Calif.

Keller, Martin B., and others. 1986. "Low Levels and Lack of Predictors of Somatotherapy and Psychotherapy Received by Depressed Patients." *Archives of General Psychiatry* 43(5): 458–66.

Kessler, Larry G. 1980. "Episodes of Psychiatric Utilization." *Medical Care* 8: 1219–27.

Kessler, Ronald C., and others. 1994. "Lifetime and Twelve-Month Prevalence of DSM-III-R Psychiatric Disorders in the United States: Results from the National Comorbidity Survey." *Archives of General Psychiatry* 51(1): 8–19.

Kupfer, David J., and others. 1992. "Five-Year Outcomes for Maintenance Therapies in Recurrent Depression." *Archives of General Psychiatry* 49: 769–73.

Lane, W. 1996. "Changing the Item Structure of the Consumer Price Index." *Monthly Labor Review* 119(12) (December): 18–25.

Newhouse, Joseph P. 1989. "Measuring Medical Prices and Understanding Their Effects." *Journal of Health Administration Education* 7(1): 19–26.

Schulberg, Herbert C., and others. 1985. "Assessing Depression in Primary Medical and Psychiatric Practices." *Archives of General Psychiatry* 42(12): 1164–70.

Scitovsky, Anne A. 1967. "Changes in the Costs of Treatment of Selected Illnesses, 1951–65." *American Economic Review* 57(5): 1182–95.

Shapiro, Matthew D., and David W. Wilcox. 1996. "Measurement in the Consumer Price Index: An Evaluation." Working Paper 5590. National Bureau of Economic Research, Cambridge, Mass. Also NBER Macroeconomics Annual 1996 (forthcoming).

U.S. Senate Finance Committee. 1996. *Final Report from the Advisory Commission to Study the Consumer Price Index*. Updated version.

Wells, Kenneth B., and others. 1994. "Use of Minor Tranquilizers and Antidepressant Medications by Depressed Outpatients: Results from the Medical Outcomes Study." *American Journal of Psychiatry* 151(5): 694–700.

Wells, Kenneth B., and others. 1996. *Caring for Depression: A RAND Study*. Harvard University Press.

Wingert, Terence D., and others. 1995. "Constructing Episodes of Care from Encounter and Claims Data: Some Methodological Issues." *Inquiry* 32: 430–43.

Comments on
Chapters 2 and 3

COMMENT BY
Dennis J. Fixler

THESE STUDIES RAISE important measurement issues, and before I discuss them I must first clarify
what is currently done in the consumer price index (CPI) regarding the
pricing of medical services.

Until January 1997 the CPI collected the prices of hospital services as
though they were separate transactions; that is, a room rate, charges for
laboratory work, and charges for other hospital services were collected
regardless of the fact that patients purchase these services within the
context of a treatment. The Bureau of Labor Statistics (BLS) has been
aware for some time of the limitations of measuring the price of hospital
services and other medical services in this manner. Accordingly, in the
late 1980s, when planning began on the producer price index (PPI) hospital index, introduced in 1993, and the physician index, introduced in
1994, the attention was directed to a treatment concept of the service
bundle to be priced. The CPI in turn adopted the use of treatment
bundles in January 1997, as described in Cardenas.[1] Because the early
indications are that this change has dampened the rate of measured price
change, the comparisons in table 2-10 of the Cutler, McClellan, and
Newhouse chapter are likely biased upward. Aside from this fact, the
comparison between the CPI and the indexes based on data from a major
teaching hospital (MTH) may not be valid; it is unclear whether the data
from the MTH were purged of Medicare data, which are out of scope for
the CPI because they are government expenditures rather than household expenditures. This matters because Catron and Murphy showed that

1. Cardenas (1996).

Medicare price inflation is low relative to measured inflation for other types of payers.[2]

My main remarks, as I said, concern the difficult measurement issues that these studies tackle. As both of them well illustrate, discussions of medical service prices necessarily involve knowledge of medicine, treatment protocols, patient characteristics, and the workings of a complex third-party payer system. Furthermore, I think it is worth noting that the United States is somewhat alone in grappling with the concept of medical services prices. In most countries, certainly European ones, there are generally no medical service market prices, as transactions are primarily with government entities and so prices are generally estimated to be at cost; hospital services, for example, largely depend on the wages of nurses and physicians. There are also differences in the market for pharmaceutical products. For example, in Sweden a single firm that in turn is owned by the government owns all retail and hospital pharmacies. The government sets drug prices according to patient characteristics—age, type of disease or handicap, and so forth. Thus the purchase of drugs by consumers is in effect a transaction with the government, but unlike in the United States, such fees are included in the Swedish CPI.

It is also worth noting that these studies make use of price data sets that are quite large relative to those used in BLS medical price indexes. The price data collected by BLS are voluntarily provided by sellers for both the CPI and the PPI, and the number of price quotes collected for each price index is determined within the framework of sampling for all the goods and service in the respective indexes. Consequently, although BLS collects monthly in the neighborhood of 100,000 prices each for the CPI and the PPI, a relatively small number of price quotes is collected for medical care services or products in each price index. In contrast, these studies used sets of patient records. To illustrate the magnitudes of difference, consider the following comparisons between the number of prices used in these studies and those used in the relevant PPI category (the comparison would be qualitatively the same with the relevant CPI category). In the PPI hospital services index for diseases and disorders of the circulatory system, the category that contains heart attack treatments, there are 161 monthly price quotes, and the PPI drug index for cardiovascular therapy contains 84 monthly quotes. Thus taken together there would be 2,940 price quotes annually. Compare this to the annual price information in the Cutler, McClellan, and Newhouse essay: 3,600 patient

2. Catron and Murphy (1996).

charges in the MTH in addition to 230,000 prices from Medicare records. For the treatment of depression, the PPI of psychiatric services, part of physician services, has 30 monthly quotes covering 11 different types of treatment, and the PPI for antidepressants contains 10 monthly quotes. Taken together there would be 480 annual quotes. The Frank, Berndt, and Busch essay has price information on 10,000 episodes parsed into 5 treatments.

The first measurement issue that I want to address concerns the utility or well-being derived from health care and the consequent application to quality adjustment. An aspect of this measurement problem is the potential gain of using outcome measures such as mortality to determine effectiveness.

The construction of accurate price indexes requires an adjustment for changes in quality. If such adjustments are not made, then one cannot decompose a price change into a pure inflation component and a non-inflationary component— a change in the nature of the good or service that justifies the price change. The production of adjustments for quality change includes three essential inputs: expert knowledge about the good, which includes its production, marketing, and nature of the transaction, quantifiable measures of the characteristics of the good, and a data set that contains these inputs. These inputs are difficult for statistical agencies to acquire in general and in medical services they are particularly elusive.

Outcome measures have received a great deal of attention as a quantifiable characteristic that may be useful in quality adjustment. As Triplett noted, the measurement of quality change in medical services can be viewed as assessing the willingness to pay for a new treatment with a new or better outcome.[3] In health care, this is done by cost-benefit analysis that often takes the form of a ratio of the treatment cost to (additional) life-year (used in Cutler, McClellan, and Newhouse) or as the ratio of treatment cost to (additional) quality adjusted life-year. The latter concept is more difficult to apply. If we are examining the cost-of-living index for a single individual, then the notion of quality of additional life-year is easy to conceptualize but difficult to measure. If, instead, we are examining the cost-of-living index for a group of individuals, each with a different reference level of well-being, then the notion of quality of additional life-year is difficult both to conceptualize and to measure.

As pointed out in the Cutler, McClellan, and Newhouse heart attack chapter, the use of mortality as an outcome is advantageous because it is

3. Triplett (1998).

dichotomous, unlike, say, the improvement in mobility after a joint replacement, which could be placed on a continuous scale. But it is an
outcome measure that has limited usefulness because it is pertinent only
for treatments that have mortality as a frequent outcome. Cutler, McClellan, and Newhouse examine the reduction in mortality as the benefit for
the increased quality resulting from the use of improved procedures, drug
therapies, and so on. This would suggest that changes in mortality rate
might be considered to be a characteristic that would influence the price
of the treatment of heart attacks. Ted Jaditz and I explicitly examined
whether the charges for heart attack treatments for a sample of Medicare
patients from New York hospitals were related to the mortality experience of the hospital relative to all hospitals in our sample. We found that
there was no relationship.[4]

The Frank, Berndt, and Busch chapter uses outcomes in a different
way—to set the benchmark level of treatment that would be considered.
Proven effectiveness based on clinical trials is used with the practice
guidelines to define the treatments and episodes to be examined. This use
avoids many thorny problems of definition, and as the authors correctly
point out, it may also lead to the exclusion of many of the treatments
provided. Standards are set as ideals and physicians are free to deviate
from them if patient characteristics warrant.

As the two cost ratios mentioned above imply, measuring the benefit
is only half the story; the measurement of the cost component is not
straightforward either. For example, in the Cutler, McClellan, and Newhouse chapter, the price of a heart attack in the cost-of-living index
(COLI) is evidently the initial hospital treatment. Elsewhere in the chapter, however, they point out that in the first year after the heart attack
there was considerable expense for hospital, physicians, and so forth. If
these are essential to the care, then should they be included in the cost?
Clearly if these additional costs were to be included in table 2-9, then the
net benefit of the additional life-years would be reduced. A proper accounting of costs requires that a more general question be answered first:
How long after the first encounter should charges be aggregated into a
single treatment charge? The answer to this question not only concerns
the proper time period for counting relevant costs but also touches on the
issue of the quality of the service. If hospitals push for early discharges,
then costs will likely go down because length of stay is an important
determinant of charges. This could bias upward any computation of net

4. Fixler and Jaditz (1997).

benefit from treatment that relied solely on the initial hospital experience. Yet because the quality of care may be reduced, the omitted future charges may in fact be higher than they otherwise would have been. In other words, there is an intertemporal tradeoff of charges, and the drawing of the boundary time period becomes important to an accurate measure of price change.

The second measurement issue concerns product classification: How should treatments be bundled and should the bundling include different types of health care providers? The pattern of technological change is such that new goods and procedures come from a variety of providers. Perhaps the best examples come from the impact that new drugs have had on hospital and physician services for the treatment of given illnesses.

There are many ways to think about the construction of product categories. In the PPI, for example, the basis for product classifications is industry production functions. In such a scheme the pharmaceutical industry is separate from physician services. The implication is that the PPI would not consider the joint psychotherapy–drug therapy in the Frank, Berndt, and Busch study unless the drug prices were part of the physician bill. In the cost-of-living sense, however, it is possible to think of consumers as switching from drugs to therapy or combining the two.

What is striking about the set of treatments for depression in the Frank, Berndt, and Busch essay is the flexibility of interpretation of the role of drugs. Taken alone, selective serotonin reuptake inhibitor drugs are substitutes for psychotherapy, whereas when paired with psychotherapy they are complements. As indicated above, such flexibility is not generally possible in the PPI, though in principle it is possible within the context of the CPI item structure because it is set by CPI staff, as described in a recent paper by Lane.[5] The hurdle to establishing such expansive item strata would be the acquisition of information about treatment paths across providers. A data source such as the insurance claim data used by Frank, Berndt, and Busch would likely be useful in this regard.

Finally, to illustrate the consequences of bundling and the method of measuring price change, suppose that I thought that only psychotherapy was the accepted treatment for depression and computed the cost as in table 3-1. Comparing the average cost in 1995 of $646 to the 1991 average cost of $924, I would find a 30 percent price decline. If I discovered my error and considered the five treatments in the table, then a simple

5. Lane (1996).

average of the costs in the PPI column of table 3-1 yields an overall treatment price decline of 35 percent. I would obtain a different answer if I instead chose any combination of the five treatments. Table 3-2 shows that the simple average of the five treatments overstates the rate of price decline and nicely demonstrates that the magnitude of the error depends on the index number formula chosen; the price reductions range from 13 to 32 percent, a rather broad range. The choice of "best" index number formula begs to be made with such information. The chained Tornqvist result, which would be close to the result one would obtain with the more common chained Fisher price index (the geometric mean of the Laspeyres and Paasche indexes), appears to be "best" because in any comparison of periods it averages the weights of importance (the shares) of each of the treatments. It thereby captures substitution between procedures. Moreover, the Tornqvist and Fisher indexes have been shown to satisfy a number of desirable properties.

COMMENT BY

Charles E. Phelps

T HESE TWO CHAPTERS—both very well constructed, and with important common elements—reveal at the same time both the value of carrying out more refined analyses of price changes through time in health care (incorporating quality adjustments) and also the difficulties and pitfalls in attempting to accomplish such analyses.

Before embarking on this discussion, it is worth reflecting on a rather central issue: Why do we want to measure price levels, and when would we want (or not) to measure changes in quality associated with price changes?[6] Figure 1 illustrates the issue when the quality of the product or service remains constant, for example, when the cost increase arises strictly from some exogenous change in the costs of producing the product (for example, higher input prices). With nominal income held constant, if the price of the good in question increases from p_1 to p_2, then consumption will fall from q_1 to q_2, and the loss in well-being—consumer surplus, formally—(to a first approximation) will be $\Delta p q_2 + .5\Delta p \Delta q$. The

6. For a sophisticated mathematical treatment of related issues, see McKenzie and Pearce (1982). The following discussion ignores a number of mathematical niceties discussed by them, but the essential ideas that follow persist in the more formalized environment of their work.

traditional Laspeyres index measures the consequences from the perspective of original consumption levels (q_1) and thus overstates the welfare loss to consumers (by ignoring that consumers will adjust quantities in response to the higher price). In figure 1 the relevant area is the rectangle A plus the two triangles B and C. Triangle C is the magnitude of overstatement of the consequences of the price increase. The Paasche index uses final consumption as the basis for analysis (rectangle A only) and thus understates the welfare consequences by ignoring the forgone consumer surplus (benefit exceeding cost—represented by triangle B) for the difference in consumption between q_1 and q_2. But, as is well known, the true welfare loss to consumers is bounded by the Paasche and Laspeyres indexes. To be clear, however, we want to know about price changes because they convey information about consumers' well-being. Higher prices make consumers worse off, with money income held constant. (This is obviously a symmetric issue regarding price declines.)

Now what do we make of a world where quality has changed? Figure 2 shows the case when the cause of the cost shift is an enhancement of quality *that is also valued by consumers*. Here the willingness to pay shifts upward at all levels of consumption, reflected in the shift from D_1 to D_2. Costs shift upward, so the equilibrium price shifts up from p_1 to p_2. The effects on consumers' well-being are now remarkably different than in the first case. In the case portrayed in figure 2, consumers are clearly better off for having the quality increase, even though price increased, since the net consumer surplus increased despite the higher cost of the good.[7] This comparison points out precisely why we need to understand quality changes in health care in order to understand the effects of price changes on consumers' well-being. If we ignore the value of higher quality, whether arriving in more effective cures or any other aspect of quality, then we may completely misunderstand the implications of a higher

7. By standard economic analysis, the measure of well-being—consumer surplus—for a representative consumer for the original quality is the sum of areas A, B, and C. Consumer surplus with the new quality is the sum of C and D. Thus well-being has increased as long as D is greater in area than A + B. The Laspeyres index would calculate a loss as areas A + B + E in this figure. The Paasche index would *add* area F to the Laspeyres measure, and Herr Paasche would probably be greatly confused to note that consumption was higher at the higher price than it was at the old lower price. Neither the Paasche nor the Laspeyres index has any way to accommodate the value of the quality improvement represented in area D. Of course, it is possible to draw figure 2 in a way to have the new quantity consumed lower than the old quantity and, indeed, to have well-being fall in response to the higher quality (if the costs of producing that higher quality exceed the value placed upon it by consumers). A perfectly functioning market would not have such a quality improvement appear, but in health care markets distorted by insurance and other subsidies, it is quite plausible to conceive of cases where quality increased in a welfare-reducing way.

Figure 1.

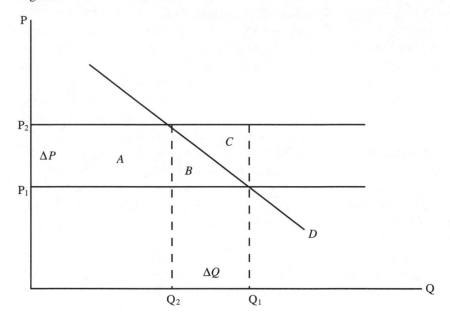

Figure 2.

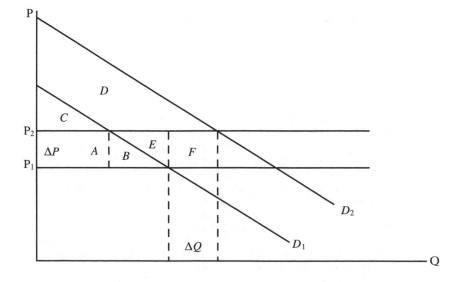

price. One of my early professors, and an early scholar in the economics of health care (Reuben Kessell, of the Graduate School of Business of the University of Chicago), used to make this point by asking the question (now slightly rephrased) "Would you rather have 1960s health care at 1960s prices or 1990s health care at 1990 prices?"

Now let me turn to the two studies of price indexes presented in this session: how can we adjust for quality of care (and its consequences for understanding the well-being of consumers), and what general implications appear? First, let me comment that the results of these two studies—if they generalize—are very dangerous to health policy analysts. We have "made our living" for the past decades by taking advantage of a well-known refrain: costs are rising in health care, probably due to the presence and growth of various distortions such as health insurance and tax subsidies to health insurance. Market forces have failed to produce a desirable equilibrium. Providers engage in a "medical arms race" that ultimately harms consumers. And so on and so forth. These two studies create a very different picture. They imply that health care costs have been falling if one takes quality improvements into account, or (put slightly differently) that consumers' well-being has systematically improved despite the appearance of higher costs in the health care sector. Dangerous stuff! These chapters imply that the fundamental premise of health policy over the past decades has possibly been fraudulent or, to put it in a more charitable light using the language of psychiatric illness suggested by one of these chapters, delusional.

Frank, Berndt, and Busch go about their analysis by looking at the costs of treating episodes of depression through time, using data from a large set of employer-based insurance claims. The period of time they examined included in it the entry of some remarkably effective new psychoactive drugs that seem to help people with depression greatly, albeit at a higher price. The authors limited their analysis to episodes of illness for which the treatment consisted of recognized protocols (for example, for psychotherapy, at least five visits; drug therapy of various intervals depending on the drug; and combinations thereof). This restricts their study to a surprisingly small fraction of all identified episodes of depression in their data (only 20–25 percent), suggesting that the vast majority of psychiatric treatment of depression does not conform to identified efficacious protocols. However, when they relax their definition of what constitutes legitimate protocols to a wider set of therapies (adding another 20–40 percent of cases treated), their fundamental results remain very similar.

   Their results are quite dramatic: the costs of treating depression fell during the period they examined (1991–95) by approximately 15–30 percent, depending on the approach taken. These results stand in sharp contrast to the producer price index components calculated by the Bureau of Labor Statistics for the same period for psychotherapeutic drugs (which showed an increase of approximately 20 percent) or the PPI index for inpatient mental illness treatment (which showed an increase of 10 percent).

   Chapter 2, by Cutler, McClellan and Newhouse, analyzes a very different illness—acute myocardial infarction (AMI, or "heart attack" in lay language)—and seeks to measure the additional benefits from improvements in treatment of AMI through time in addition to measuring costs. They do this by looking at one single dimension of improvement—survival—and valuing additional life-years at $25,000 per life-year. (They note that this probably understates the value of improved survival but carried out the analysis with this conservative approach to emphasize their point. I will return to an implication for understanding the time path of consumer well-being associated with cost and survival changes.)

   As with the chapter on the costs of treating depression, this chapter finds that the quality-adjusted cost of treating major heart disease has fallen through time, taking quality improvements into account. Whereas CPI and related indexes showed *real* (extra GDP deflator) increases of 2.4–3.4 percent per year, they estimate that the cost-of-living index (here, literally, since they are estimating the costs of surviving a heart attack) fell by about 1 percent per year over the 1984–91 period.

   These two chapters illuminate the importance of understanding quality of care improvements, but they also point out, either directly or indirectly, some of the hazards of attempting to do so. Let me point out some of these issues, not intending these as derogatory remarks about these chapters, but rather to use their work as the basis for understanding the difficulty of carrying out quality adjustments appropriately.

   1. *Understanding the true marginal benefits of new therapies.* Particularly in chapter 2, the authors have admirably used data from controlled clinical trials to understand the health effects of various therapies (see table 2-6). Yet these clinical studies seldom estimate the appropriate marginal benefits of one therapy on top of another. Available studies allowed the estimation of the effects of some combinations of therapies. (Their "upper" and "lower" estimates account for such interactions.) Yet the literature does not support an understanding of the consequences of many combinations of these therapies, and their own analysis suggests

that most of the cost increase through time has been associated with increases in the intensity of treatment. This remains a risk in all such studies as these. Does the estimate of benefit take into account other therapies that might also have been provided to the patient? The costs of those therapies appear in the usual "cost-of-treatment" measures (at least when well conducted), but the benefits may be overstated.

The consequences for understanding the time path of consumer net benefit depend on whether the passage of time brings more or fewer "stacked" therapies. If, as the Cutler, McClellan, and Newhouse analysis suggests, treatment intensity is increasing through time, then it seems plausible that the frequency of "stacked" treatments will also increase, and the incremental benefits of second, third, and subsequent treatments may be significantly less than the benefits of those same treatments applied as the initial therapy. This could cause an overstatement of the increase in benefits through time and hence an understatement of the increases in net costs through time.

2. *Omitted measures of benefit.* The AMI study uses only the benefits from improved mortality as a measure of benefit. Other studies have shown that benefits in other areas (improved functional status, freedom from chest pain, and so on) arise with increased treatment rates.[8] The omission of such dimensions of value biases upward the apparent net costs of treatment by omitting some benefits. The consequences for understanding the time path of net costs depend on whether the amount of such unmeasured benefit increases or decreases through time. This is exactly analogous to the generic issue of whether one measures anything about quality of care at all. If (as I suspect) treatment for AMI began by applying therapies to the most seriously ill patients and then extended them to those less seriously ill through time, then the improvements in health in areas other than mortality will grow faster than the improvements in mortality, and the omission of some aspects of benefit will bias the apparent net cost path (through time) upward.

3. *Shifts toward the treatment frontier.* The Frank, Berndt, and Busch chapter emphasizes the importance of knowing how much treatment is "off the frontier" of "best practice" at any point in time. In their study of treatment of depression, up to 80 percent of treatment was "off the frontier," although another 20–40 percent was "close." They did not provide any estimate of the time path of these ratios. It should be clear, however, that if the time path shows movement toward the treatment

8. See Mark and others (1994).

efficacy frontier, then more net benefit should occur through time for the same expenditure of resources, and any estimate of the net cost increase through time will contain an upward bias.

The literature on this issue is quite disturbing. We know from cross-sectional studies that there is widespread disagreement about the proper ways to use medical therapies of almost any type.[9] One's chances of receiving a particular therapy can vary by an order of magnitude for many treatments, depending on where one lives. This issue, described in the medical care literature as the "medical practice variations" problem, has been studied extensively by physicians, epidemiologists, and a few economists. The economic consequences of these variations are large,[10] indeed, larger than the usual "welfare loss" issues normally studied by economists,[11] at least according to one comparison.[12] These widely varying patterns of treatment require that a substantial fraction of therapy is not on the efficient frontier.

The extent to which this matters, and the potential for important change through time (which is the key issue in understanding effects on price index measures through time) varies greatly by type of therapy. For example, studies of hospitalization for AMI show that regional patterns of treatment have a very low coefficient of variation (COV) of 0.1, implying a strong agreement about when to use hospitalization. Use of coronary artery bypass graft and percutaneous transluminal angioplasty (or more commonly, "balloon angioplasty") have COV measures of 0.3 to 0.4, showing greater disagreement about when to use the therapies, and hence greater risk that some of the treatment is not on the efficient frontier. Hospitalizations for psychiatric illnesses, however, have very large COV measures (0.6 or higher), suggesting even greater disagreement about the proper use of therapy, and hence still greater risk of nonfrontier use of the therapy. It seems plausible that the time path would show migration toward the efficient frontier, but historical data on this are not particularly encouraging (in the sense that when repeated measures of variability have been made at different times, the coefficients of variation do not seem to collapse much). If there is movement toward the frontier, then (as noted before) the time series analysis of net benefits and costs must adjust for this somehow to capture fully the improvement in benefits through time.

9. See Phelps and Mooney (1993); Phelps (1992); Phelps (forthcoming) for further discussion.
10. Phelps and Parente (1989); Phelps and Mooney (1992).
11. For example, Arrow (1963); Pauly (1986); Zeckhauser (1970).
12. Phelps (forthcoming).

I might add that the encroachment of managed care will likely—if anything—increase the proportion of care delivered that is on or near the efficient frontier, since these organizations (at least when paid on a capitation or similar basis) have strong financial incentives to move toward the efficient frontier.

4. *The value of benefits will change through time.* The Cutler, McClellan, and Newhouse chapter uses a fixed rate of $25,000 per life-year produced as the incremental value. In a society with steadily growing income, this causes a systematic understatement of the time path of benefits, and hence an overstatement of the rate of change of net costs of therapy. The logic of this is fairly simple: when we have more money, we can consume better wine, buy finer stereos and more comfortable cars, and play golf on more interesting golf courses than when we have less money. Thus the value of adding a year of life is greater when we have higher incomes. In the United States, real per capita income increases at about 1–2 percent per year over the long haul. Garber and Phelps show that the value of adding a life-year rises systematically with increased income (they suggest a rule of thumb based on a wide variety of studies that the value of a life-year saved is about twice annual income).[13] The overall effect on the apparent time path of net costs of a therapy can thus be considerable, and the direction of bias is quite clear. When income rises through time, using a constant value of quality-adjusted life-years will cause the apparent rate of net cost increase to be too high over time.

5. *The mix of patients studied may change through time.* Studies such as the two discussed here gain much of their insight from following populations through time using extant databases, often insurance claims. As we pursue such studies in the future, we must carefully attend to the mix of people enrolled in the underlying health plans (or whatever the source of the data). Health plan data are not a carefully controlled panel following the same individuals through time; they represent, rather, a time series of cross-sections of the population, cross-sections that can readily change in many ways. If such shifts in the populations studied affect the propensity of the individuals to have the illness being studied, or the severity of such illnesses, then there is an obvious risk of distortion, with no necessary direction of bias in terms of understanding the time path of quality-adjusted price changes. The chapter by Frank, Berndt, and Busch uses data from private insurance plans where the issue of

13. Garber and Phelps (1997).

patient migration and selection can possibly loom large. The Cutler, McClellan, and Newhouse chapter relies on combinations of data, some using the entire Medicare population, and some using carefully controlled clinical studies where the entry criteria for eligibility in the study are quite explicit. However, it would seem desirable to always attend to the issues of selection, patient mix, and the like, when undertaking the types of studies necessary to understand the time path of quality-adjusted price changes in health care.

Conclusion

We get a very different picture of the costs of treating illnesses when we use the types of approaches such as these two chapters employ than when we use producer price index types of measures that fail to adjust for changes in quality of care. In the two cases studied here, the implications as to how well the health care system has been performing are the reverse of the usual conclusion: rather than showing relentless cost growth (the usual conclusion), these chapters both show that quality-adjusted price indicators have fallen over recent years. I might note that this result does not automatically obtain. In an analysis of the time path of antibiotic prices presented in chapter 4, the efficacy of a given drug in combating bacterial infections will almost certainly fall through time due to increased resistance of the bacteria to the effects of the drug.[14] How much these results generalize to other areas of the health care sector remains to be seen, but the consequences for public policy are great if they generalize even only partly. Rather than confronting markets that seem to be running amok, we may need to think about health care markets (as we do personal computers and related markets) as sectors of the economy marked by considerable technical innovation, increasing productivity in the underlying goal of improving health of the public, and—after taking such improvements into account—as markets where prices are falling, not rising. Remarkable!

References

Arrow, Kenneth J. 1963. "Uncertainty and the Welfare Economics of Medical Care." *American Economic Review* 53(5): 943–73.
Cardenas, Elaine. 1996. "Revision of the CPI Hospital Services Component." *Monthly Labor Review* 119(12) (December): 40–48.

14. Phelps (1989).

Catron, Brian, and Bonnie Murphy. 1996. "Hospital Price Inflation: What Does the New PPI Tell Us?" *Monthly Labor Review* (July): 24–31.

Fixler, D., and T. Jaditz. 1997. "Hedonic Adjustment of Hospital Service Price Inflation: An Application to Medicare Prices." BLS Working Paper 299.

Garber, Alan M., and Charles E. Phelps. 1997. "The Economic Foundations of Cost-Effectiveness Analysis." *Journal of Health Economics* 16(1): 1–31.

Lane, W. 1996. "Changing the Item Structure of the Consumer Price Index." *Monthly Labor Review* 119(12) (December): 18–25.

Mark, Daniel B., and others. 1994. "Use of Medical Resources and Quality of Life after Acute Myocardial Infarction in Canada and the United States." *New England Journal of Medicine* 331(17): 1130–35.

McKenzie, George W., and Ivor F. Pearce. 1982. "Welfare Analysis: A Synthesis." *American Economic Review* 72(4): 669–82.

Pauly, Mark V. 1986. "Taxation, Health Insurance, and Market Failure in the Medical Economy." *Journal of Economic Literature* 24(2): 629–75.

Phelps, Charles E. 1989. "Bug/Drug Resistance: Sometimes Less Is More." *Medical Care* 29(2) (February): 194–203.

———. 1992. "Diffusion of Information in Medical Care." *Journal of Economic Perspectives* 6(3) (Summer): 23–42.

———. In press. "The Role of Information in the Supply and Demand of Health Care." In *Handbook of Health Economics*, edited by Joseph P. Newhouse and Anthony Culyer. Amsterdam: North Holland.

Phelps, Charles E., and Cathleen Mooney. 1992. "Correction and Update on Priority Setting in Medical Technology Assessment in Medical Care." *Medical Care* 31(8) (August): 744–745.

———. 1993. "Variations in Medical Practice Use: Causes and Consequences." In *Competitive Approaches to Health Care Reform*, edited by Richard J. Arnould, Robert F. Rich, and William D. White. Washington, D.C.: Urban Institute Press.

Phelps, Charles E., and Stephen T. Parente. 1990. "Priority Setting in Medical Technology and Medical Practice Assessment." *Medical Care* 29(8) (August): 703–23.

Triplett, Jack E. 1998. "What's Different about Health? Human Repair and Car Repair in the National Accounts." Brookings Institution.

Zeckhauser, Richard J. 1970. "Medical Insurance: A Case Study of the Tradeoff between Risk Spreading and Appropriate Incentives." *Journal of Economic Theory* 2(1): 10–26.

4

The Economics
of Antibiotics: An
Exploratory Study

Sara Fisher Ellison and
Judith K. Hellerstein

A NTIBIOTICS ARE ARGUABLY the most effective class of drugs ever developed. Before the advent of antibiotics, bacterial infections such as tuberculosis and pneumonia were leading killers of adults, and children routinely died of such bacterial infectious diseases as tuberculosis, meningitis, pertussis (whooping cough), scarlet fever, and rheumatic fever. The introduction of penicillin in clinical use in the 1940s marked the beginning of our ability to fight bacterial infections. During the 1950s and 1960s, the development of amoxicillin, erythromycin, tetracycline, cephalosporins, and other broad spectrum antibiotics furthered this process, as has the more recent development of other broad spectrum antibiotics such as fluoroquinolones. Antibiotics, together with advances in vaccines against some bacterial infections, have significantly reduced childhood morbidity and mortality. Indeed, of the above-listed childhood diseases, only meningitis continues to be a real threat to children in the United States.

Antibiotics differ from other prescription drugs in their pharmacological characteristics, of course, as well as in their regulatory treatment and in the way demand for their use arises. All of these factors contribute to explaining today's market structure for antibiotics, one with many unusual characteristics that distinguish it from the market structures for other pharmaceuticals. In particular, as we argue in detail below, incen-

We thank Ernst Berndt, Tom Croghan, Patricia Danzon, Richard Frank, Henry Grabowski, and Jack Triplett for helpful comments, and Lori Melichar for research assistance. This work was funded by a grant from Eli Lilly through the National Bureau of Economic Research.

tives for pharmaceutical companies to innovate and develop new antibiotics are different from incentives to develop drugs that do not treat infectious diseases.

In this chapter, we contribute two main findings that may differ from the conventional wisdom about antibiotics. First, we conduct a detailed analysis of wholesale price growth over the last decade in one large class of antibiotics. As part of this analysis, we consider how wholesale prices have differed across various retail markets to which they are sold in order to get a sense of how the changing market for pharmaceuticals may be affecting prices. We also compare our price indexes to the comparable official government price index for the class of antibiotics that we consider. Our main finding is that prices have been growing very slowly even in nominal terms, much more slowly than official government statistics suggest. This should be good news for consumers of antibiotics.

Second, we consider how innovation of new antibiotics may be affected by the growth of antibiotic-resistant bacteria. We demonstrate that because of drug resistance, innovation of new antibiotics may be less than would be optimal for society in a way that has not previously been demonstrated. So although the fact that prices of existing antibiotics have not been increasing over the last decade is good news for consumers, the growth of drug resistance and its impact on innovation may be bad news.

Institutional Facts about Antibiotics

Antibiotics are different from other prescription drugs along many dimensions, all of which affect the various competitive aspects of this market including pricing and research and development. First, the Food and Drug Administration approval process for antibiotics is different from that for other drugs. Approvals for new and generic antibiotics have always been granted by a different branch of the FDA than have those for other drugs. Because the production process for early antibiotics essentially was as easy as following a recipe, the FDA was not as concerned with quality control for generic antibiotics as it was with other classes of drugs.[1] As a result, approval for generic antibiotics has always been reasonably easy to obtain. This situation, coupled with the fact that some early antibiotics never had patent protection, has resulted in higher market penetration of generic antibiotics relative to other types of

---

1. See Hellerstein (1995) for more on the FDA approval process for antibiotics.

drugs.[2] In addition to price competition resulting from generic penetration, there may also be price competition across different types of antibiotics, since many different antibiotics are often indicated for use against the same bacteria. Evidence on this is somewhat weak, however.[3]

The efficacy and success of antibiotics also set them apart from other drugs. Before the advent of antibiotics, bacterial infections such as tuberculosis, pneumonia, and typhoid fever were leading killers of people worldwide. By the mid-1980s, however, these infections either were cured easily by readily available (and inexpensive) antibiotics or had been virtually eradicated in the developed world. The success of antibiotics was so great that the public largely believed the war against bacterial infections had been won. It is not surprising, then, that public and government attention has focused on more contemporary killers, such as AIDS and cancer. Moreover, with perceived fierce generic price competition and the impressive efficacy of inexpensive and effective antibiotics, it is equally unsurprising that pharmaceutical manufacturers may have found little reason recently to allocate scarce R&D resources to the development of antibiotics.

It is difficult to obtain direct or indirect empirical evidence on how incentives to pharmaceutical companies to invest in R&D in antibiotics have changed. An informal telephone survey of major U.S. and Japanese pharmaceutical companies conducted during a workshop sponsored by the National Institutes of Health found that half of the firms had reduced or completely phased out research on antibiotics.[4] This is not to say that no research is being done. Some companies have been reported to be beginning new research initiatives to combat the problem of resistant bacteria.[5] Data from the FDA for the past thirteen years show no discernible trend in approvals of new antibiotics, but the sample sizes are small—the average number of approvals per year is two. Moreover, with the lag in time from the beginning of development of a drug to its eventual FDA approval, it is not clear what time frame to consider when thinking about how innovation has changed.

Pricing Patterns

Long-term price trends are one of the most important features to consider when examining the economics of antibiotics. The last decade

---

2. Hellerstein (1995).
3. Ellison and others (1997).
4. Tomasz (1994).
5. "Drug Makers Go All out to Squash 'Superbugs'" (1996).

has been a particularly interesting one for pharmaceuticals in general and antibiotics in particular. The most important and salient change over this period has probably been the phenomenal restructuring of health care in this country with a marked shift toward managed care.[6] Whereas in the mid-1980s relatively few patients had outpatient insurance coverage of pharmaceuticals, managed care drug benefits of one type or another have become increasingly prevalent. As pharmaceuticals have been increasingly included in patients' benefit packages, much of the decisionmaking about the type of prescription written and dispensed has shifted from the physician and patient to the managed care company. In addition to managed care growth, there has been some change in this period in state laws requiring pharmacists to dispense lower-priced generic versions of drugs. Finally, there has been growing public awareness of antibiotic resistance over the past two or three years. With these changes in mind, we examine prices across different types of manufacturers and across different markets, or "channels of distribution," to get a better sense of whether these changes may lead to changes in the competitive structure of the antibiotics market.

The retail price of a course of an antibiotic to treat a typical adult bacterial infection ranges from around $10 for generic amoxicillin, an old off-patent antibiotic, to around $50 for Zithromax, a new on-patent antibiotic, and around $80 for Ceclor, the branded version of cefaclor, a drug that only recently went off patent and has a very complicated and expensive manufacturing process. A course of generic cefaclor sells for around $55. We do not have any information on the extent of markups in antibiotics. Even with information on marginal costs, it is difficult to know whether and how to account for the large fixed costs of R&D when calculating markups. Perhaps the best way, then, to decide whether antibiotics are inexpensive (relative to their value to consumers) is to note the willingness of physicians and patients to use antibiotics inappropriately. For example, one study reports that in a careful analysis of the impacts of health insurance on utilization, approximately 16 percent of antibiotics prescriptions filled were indicated for treating viral infections, where there is no evidence that they are effective.[7] Moreover, this occurred frequently even in cases when patients had to pay copayments for their prescription drugs, so people are willing to pay for antibiotics that may not help them.

6. "A Shift of Power in Pharmaceuticals" (1994); "The Changing Environment for U.S. Pharmaceuticals" (1993).
7. Newhouse and Insurance Experiment Group (1993).

In order to calculate price indexes, we use two data sets. Our first data set, collected by IMS America, contains wholesale quantities and revenues of all prescription antibiotics sold in the United States from October 1985 to December 1991. These quantities and revenues are those from transactions between manufacturers or distributors and two separate groups of retailers: hospitals and retail pharmacies. The data are at the level of presentation for each pharmaceutical product.[8] Our second data set, also collected by IMS America, has a similar structure but covers the months September 1990 through August 1996. The other main difference is that after January 1992 the data in this second set are divided into a richer group of retailers, or channels of distribution: federal facilities, clinics, HMOs, nonfederal facilities, chain drugstores, independent drugstores, food stores, and long-term care.[9] Note that the definition of "hospitals" in the first data set corresponds closely to that of "nonfederal facilities" in the second and that "retail pharmacies" corresponds to the sum of "independent drugstores," "chain drugstores," and "food stores."

We examine in detail price growth in one important subclass of antibiotics, cephalosporins.[10] The first cephalosporin, cephalexin, was introduced by Eli Lilly in 1971 under the brand name Keflex. Other so-called first generation cephalosporins, such as cefadroxil and cephradine, entered soon thereafter. Now in existence are second and third generation cephalosporins, so classified because of similarities in their molecular structures. Our data sets contain a total of twenty-four chemically distinct cephalosporins.

We focus on cephalosporins for a number of reasons. First, it is a large and important subclass of antibiotics. For example, over the six years ending in August 1996, cephalosporins comprised approximately 40 percent of total revenues of antibiotics in the United States.[11] Second, it is a subclass of antibiotics that is active against a wide range of bacteria, indicated for a wide range of infections, used in many different clinical settings, and sold in all different channels of distribution. Given this, we

8. A presentation is a particular choice of packaging and dose-form for a product, for example, 150 mg coated tablets in bottles of 100, or 25 ml of 5 percent aqueous solution in a vial for intravenous injection. A drug will often be sold in many presentations simultaneously.

9. Note that the category for HMOs only includes prescriptions dispensed at HMO-owned hospitals and pharmacies, not prescriptions dispensed elsewhere but paid for by an HMO drug benefit. The HMO channel of distribution, then, reflects only a small portion of the influence that HMOs and other managed care have had on pharmaceutical purchasing.

10. The name is derived from the Greek island of Cephalos, where antibiotic activity was observed in isolates from shellfish.

11. Authors' calculation.

can examine pricing patterns in all channels of distribution from which IMS collects data and be fairly confident that our findings for cephalosporins are not special to a particular clinical or market setting. In addition, cephalosporins are a group of drugs in which innovating manufacturers are quite important, in part because cephalosporins are among the newer antibiotics (relative to, say, penicillins), but have also been subject to generic entry. Finally, cephalosporins is a subclass that has been analyzed in the economics literature previously.[12]

To look at broad pricing patterns, we need to aggregate over the thousands of products for which we have data. We do this by computing monthly price indexes where the index is calculated as the weighted sum of price changes for all presentations sold in a month. In particular, we compute Tornqvist price indexes using as weights the average revenue share of each presentation in the two months for which we calculate the price change.[13] Tornqvist indexes have the advantage (over, for example, traditional fixed-weight Laspeyres indexes) that the weights are allowed to vary from month to month as different drugs lose or gain relative importance in the market. In addition, new drugs can enter the price index in their second month, which is the first month for which one can compute a price change.

Price indexes usually start at one in the first month of the data, but we are interested not just in price growth over the period of our two data sets but also in differences in the levels of prices across the different channels of distribution. We therefore normalize our price indexes to reflect relative price differences across markets. For example, in the first data set, which begins in October 1985, we start the price index for cephalosporins sold to hospitals at a base price of 1.00, but we normalize the pharmacy price index to start at a base price of 1.26. To compute this figure of 1.26, we calculate a weighted sum of the price ratios of all the presentations sold to both pharmacies and hospitals. The weights are total revenues (in pharmacies and hospitals) of each presentation as a share of the total across all identical presentations. As our results show, normalizing the

---

12. See, for example, Griliches and Cockburn (1994); Ellison and others (1997).

13. The Tornqvist price index calculated for N products in a month t is

$$I_t = \exp\left(\sum_{n-1}^{N} \overline{s_{nt}} \log\left(\frac{P_{nt}}{P_{nt-1}}\right)\right) I_{t-1},$$

where P_{nt} is the price of the nth product in month t, $\overline{s_{nt}} = 0.5(s_{nt} + s_{nt-1})$, Q is quantity, and

$$s_{nt} = \frac{P_{nt}Q_{nt}}{\sum_{n=1}^{N} P_{nt}Q_{nt}}.$$

indexes in this way is important to understanding the pricing patterns of wholesale cephalosporins.

Figure 4-1 contains the summary findings of our price index calculations. We calculate an overall Tornqvist price index for all cephalosporins and compare our index to the official producer price index for cephalosporins. We find an overall annual average growth rate (AAGR) of prices for cephalosporins over the period January 1988 to August 1996 of 0.76 percent. (We report the index over this period because the Bureau of Labor Statistics [BLS] only started computing a producer price index for cephalosporins in January 1988.) Note also from the figure a pronounced fall of the index over more recent months.

The AAGR of the BLS official producer price index for cephalosporins over this period is markedly different at 4.54 percent.[14] These basic results are consistent with other literature addressing upward biases in the BLS's price index calculations for pharmaceuticals.[15] By virtually any standard, the increase we find in the price of cephalosporins is modest and suggests that there have been significant competitive pressures to keep price increases low over this period.[16]

There are three possible reasons why our price index for cephalosporins differs so dramatically from the official BLS price index.[17] First, our index incorporates new products immediately, whereas the BLS only does so every four to seven years.[18] Second, our index allows for changing weights to reflect changing revenue shares of products. Third, our data are a near census of sales made by both manufacturers and distributors, whereas the BLS uses only a sample of products, and that sample is only from production facilities.

A formal examination of the BLS price index for cephalosporins is beyond the scope of this chapter.[19] Although we cannot mimic the BLS's

14. Even the official rate of overall inflation as reflected in the consumer price index over this period was much higher than our figure, with an AAGR of 3.55 percent.

15. Baye, Maness, and Wiggins (1990); Berndt, Griliches, and Rosett (1993); and Griliches and Cockburn (1994).

16. We have not completed as comprehensive a study of the prices of other antibiotics, but computation of a general price index for each of penicillin, erythromycin, trimethoprim, and chloramphenicol suggests similarly slow price growth.

17. For a summary of the BLS's procedures in calculating the producer price index, see *BLS Handbook of Methods* (1997).

18. During our sample period, the BLS resampled pharmaceutical products over the course of 1987 and again over 1992. Recently, the BLS adopted a procedure to incorporate generics into the price index when they first enter the market. For a summary of this procedure and information on the timing of the introductions of new goods into the PPI for Prescription Pharmaceuticals, see Kanoza (1996).

19. For an analysis of this kind, see Berndt, Griliches, and Rosett (1993).

Figure 4-1. *All Cephalosporins Price Indexes*

January 1988 = 1.0

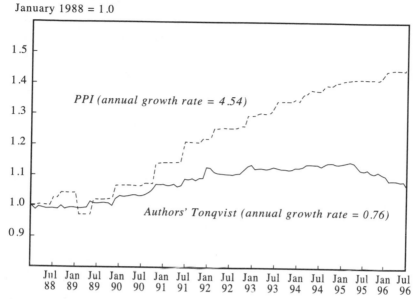

Source: Authors' calculations and various reports published by the Bureau of Labor Statistics.

Laspeyres index methods exactly, we did attempt to mimic BLS procedures in a variety of ways. First, we calculated a modified Tornqvist index, where we incorporated new products only when the BLS did (rather than instantaneously). For this price index, we calculate an AAGR of 1.45 percent from January 1988 to August 1996. We also calculated a fixed-weight Laspeyres index, but again allowed new products to enter when the BLS did. For this index, we obtain a very similar AAGR over this period of 1.39 percent. These alternative price indexes have AAGRs that are somewhat above the AAGR of our preferred Tornqvist index, but still far below the BLS's AAGR of 4.54 percent.[20] Therefore, we suspect that most of the difference between our Tornqvist index and the BLS index is due to sampling issues in the choice of products used to construct the BLS index rather than issues related to the frequency of resampling or the adjustment of weights over time. This is

20. On a related note, this exercise implies that differences in price growth between older and newer cephalosporins over the time period of our sample has not been substantial (at least in revenue-weighted terms). Of course, our index does not tackle the "new goods" problem. This is the difficult problem of adjusting for differences in quality-adjusted relative prices of new drugs versus old drugs; our index only captures revenue weighted price growth of existing drugs. For more on this question, see Griliches and Cockburn (1994).

similar to the conclusion of a related study that attributes approximately half of the difference between their Tornqvist index for prescription pharmaceuticals and the BLS index (from January 1984 to December 1989) to sampling problems in the BLS sample.[21]

Figure 4-2 contains information on price indexes we computed separately for cephalosporins sold to hospitals and pharmacies. We combine both of our data sets and report a price index over the entire period from October 1985 through August 1996.[22] The price index for sales to hospitals is normalized to begin at a base price of 1 at the beginning of the period, with the price of sales to pharmacies normalized to a higher level (1.26) to reflect differences in relative prices across the two channels.

The striking feature of figure 4-2 is that the prices of cephalosporins sold to drugstores were higher than those sold to hospitals at the beginning of our data and this gap widened over most of the last decade. In fact, hospital prices have been falling slowly but fairly steadily over the period. This is consistent with increased formulary use in hospitals and the resulting downward pressure on drug prices as hospitals bargain with pharmaceutical companies. At the end of our data pharmacy prices do fall, so it is possible that the trend of widening price differentials across the two channels of distribution is beginning to reverse itself. This is consistent, of course, with recent increased bargaining power by pharmacies. It is also consistent with the increasing pressures of managed care to keep prices of drugs sold in pharmacies low and with public pressure over the last few years to reduce prices. We provide further evidence on this below when we disaggregate the data by finer channels of distribution.

Table 4-1 and figure 4-3 exploit the richer data on channels of distribution that we have in the data since 1992. We compute separate indexes for each of the eight channels. The price of cephalosporins sold to "hospitals" (nonfederal facilities) is normalized to begin at 1 at the beginning of 1992; indexes for sales to other channels are normalized to begin at levels relative to that of hospitals. There is notable variation both in the

21. Berndt, Griliches, and Rosett (1993). We cannot construct a price index for sales made by manufacturers only, which would represent the price index that the BLS sampling methods try to capture. We doubt that the prices of sales by manufacturers have been growing more quickly than sales by distributors, since as we show below, the growth rates of prices of drugs sold to hospitals and chain drugstores are below that of other channels of distribution. We expect that bigger purchasers such as hospitals and chain drugstores are more likely, not less likely, to purchase directly from manufacturers.

22. The new data are linked to the old data at the midpoint of where they overlap, April 1991. We confirmed that during the period in which the old and new data overlap, the pricing patterns are very similar across the two data sets.

Figure 4-2. *Cephalosporins Price Indexes*

Hospitals, October 1985 = 1.0

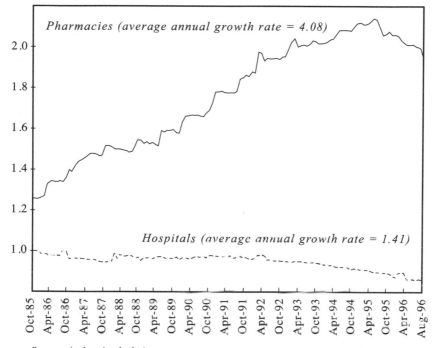

Source: Authors' calculations.

Table 4-1. *Cephalosporins Average Annual Growth Rates, January 1992–August 1996*

Channel of distribution	Growth rate (percent)	Average monthly revenue (millions of dollars)	Base price
Chain stores	−0.90	72.2	1.08
Independents	0.31	45.4	1.10
Clinics	−0.75	3.7	1.07
Food stores	0.40	15.2	1.12
HMOs	2.60	2.9	0.98
Long-term care	1.52	5.2	1.03
Nonfederal facilities	−2.68	78.9	1.00
Federal facilities	−5.41	2.7	1.01

Source: Authors' calculations.

Figure 4-3. *Cephalosporins Price Indexes*

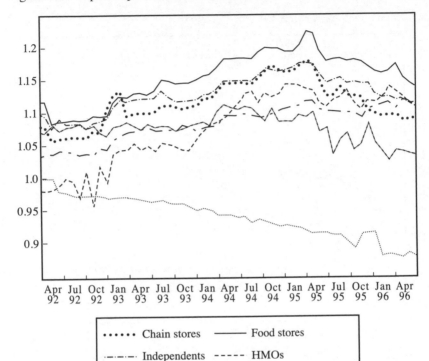

Source: Authors' calculations.

levels of prices and their growth rates across channels.[23] The biggest channels of distribution (in terms of revenue) continue to be nonfederal facilities, and the segment of the pharmacy sector represented by chain drugstores. Of course, the pricing patterns across these two channels of distribution look very similar to those we report in figure 4-2 for the same period.[24] Interestingly, the index for cephalosporins sold to independent

23. In figure 4-3, we omit the price index for sales to federal facilities. Prices have been falling dramatically in that small market, and including that price index obscures differences across the other bigger, more interesting channels. Summary statistics on sales to federal facilities do appear in table 4-1.

24. We note that these diverging price indexes are *not* a function of the changing mix of products used in hospitals versus other channels of distribution. When we compute price indexes for only those products sold in hospitals and in each other channel of distribution at the beginning of the period, the price index patterns are very similar.

drugstores closely follows that of chain drugstores, with the exceptions that independent drugstore prices start higher than prices to chains and have fallen recently by less than prices to chain drugstores. The trend in price growth for sales to food stores is similar to that of independent drugstores, but the level of prices is generally slightly higher. Prices to clinics tend also to move with those of independent drugstores but remain at lower levels throughout the period.

Perhaps the most interesting pattern in figure 4-3 is that of HMOs. Prices of cephalosporins sold to HMOs were lower in January 1992 than those sold to any other channel of distribution, but they experienced by far the largest AAGR (2.6 percent), placing HMO prices in the middle of the pack by August 1996.

The patterns reflected in figure 4-3 make it clear that both the level and growth of prices of cephalosporins sold are quite different across finely defined channels of distribution. The fact that prices to chain drugstores have fallen more recently than prices to food stores or independent drugstores is most consistent with increased bargaining power of chain drugstores relative to other types of drugstores. This may, in turn, be partially a function of pressure by managed care companies to reduce prices charged by chain pharmacies with which these companies often contract, pressure that gets transmitted to the wholesale level. The fact that HMO prices start low but experience the steepest AAGR over this period is consistent with the anecdote we hear of large price concessions being given to HMOs a few years ago coupled with a more recent retreat from this practice. The reason for this may be that HMO pharmacies have not become as prevalent as might have been expected a few years ago; today most HMOs have patients fill prescriptions at retail establishments like chainstore pharmacies.

The richness of our data sets allows us to characterize the level and growth of prices of cephalosporins sold to different channels of distribution. These results suggest that the interaction of supply and demand has a measurable effect on relative prices across channels of distribution. The most salient feature of these indexes is the relatively slow growth rate of prices of sales across *all* channels of distribution.

Price changes themselves cannot lead one to draw firm conclusions about the extent to which pharmaceutical manufacturers are making profits on the sale of cephalosporins. This is particularly true in a market like pharmaceuticals, where it is difficult to account for the high research and development costs when analyzing profits. Nonetheless, the fact that prices have been rising only slowly and appear to be rising most slowly in markets where buyers have bargaining power suggests that, absent dramatic cost decreases of which we are not aware, profit margins for cephalosporins are declining in real terms and may continue to decline as health care markets continue to consolidate. Consumers should perceive this as one positive by-product of market consolidation in health care. Antibiotics, however, may not remain inexpensive and effective forever.

The Public Health and Economic Implications of Antibiotics Use

The very nature of infectious diseases, such as those treated with antibiotics, results in interesting economic and public health characteristics of the use of antibiotics. In particular, there is a positive externality associated with the use of antibiotics. The benefits of an individual's consumption of an antibiotic do not accrue solely to the patient consuming it. One person's consumption of an antibiotic benefits others because it reduces the probability that others will contract the bacterial infection. One result of this positive externality is that one cannot measure the social benefit of antibiotics simply by summing up the benefits that accrue privately to individuals when they consume antibiotics. If an individual's decision to consume an antibiotic is based solely on the private benefits of consuming that antibiotic, the individual will demand too little of that antibiotic relative to what would be optimal for society. Therefore, overall market demand for the antibiotic will be artificially low relative to the social optimum. If demand is too low, prices may be lower than what they would be in the absence of these positive externalities. If prices of antibiotics are too low relative to the social optimum, this could create conditions where the incentives for private pharmaceutical firms to develop new antibiotics will be lower than they would be in the absence of positive externalities.

There are a couple of caveats to the magnitude and effects of these positive externalities. First, to the extent that the decisionmaker for the consumption of antibiotics may be the physician rather than the patient, overall market demand will be determined by physicians' preferences. If physicians care about infection transmission, they may incorporate the positive externality of antibiotics use into their decisions, which may mitigate the problem. To our knowledge, there is no evidence on how the existence of externalities actually affects decisions made by physicians. Second, even if demand for antibiotics is too low, prices may not be lower than socially optimal for two reasons. First, if the market is so competitive that no economic profits are being realized on the sale of pharmaceuticals, prices will be equal to marginal costs no matter what demand is. In this case, however, there is no incentive to innovate and develop new antibiotics since pharmaceutical manufacturers need to be able to set prices above marginal costs in order to recoup the large R&D costs of new drug development. Second and perhaps more important, there are reasons why in the absence of positive externalities prices may be too high relative to the social optimum, so the positive externalities may actually correct this problem. This could occur if, for example, patients' or physicians' private valuation of aspects of antibiotics such as their broad-spectrum capabilities are higher than social valuation. We return to these points below.

Unfortunately, there are also negative externalities associated with the use of antibiotics. Each use of a given antibiotic increases the probability that a particular bacterial strain will become resistant to that antibiotic, and indeed, given that resistance can be spread across genetically differ- ent bacteria, each use of a given antibiotic against a particular bacterium increases the probability that other bacterial strains will become resistant to it. Infectious disease specialists and public health officials have sounded warnings about the perils of drug resistance for years, but these warnings have rarely made it into the public consciousness, or the consciousness of health care practitioners, until recently.[25] Pharmaceutical manufacturers have traditionally responded to drug resistance by altering existing antibi- otics subtly in ways that thwart resistance temporarily and that may not have been costly to develop. Over time, however, even these new genera- tions of drugs have become ineffectual against certain resistant bacterial strains. As a result of this negative externality, the private demand for antibiotics exceeds what would be socially optimal if individuals properly internalized the social cost of antibiotics use. This is the main social cost associated with "overprescription of antibiotics," where antibiotics are prescribed inappropriately (for example, for viral infections).

Recently, the press has reported on three cases, in Japan, Michigan, and New Jersey, of a strain of staphylococcus aureus that showed an intermediate level of resistance to vancomycin.[26] Such reports are of par- ticular concern because vancomycin is considered the "last resort" antibi- otic for staph infections, for use when a bacterium has proved resistant to all other antibiotics. No strain of staph had before developed resistance to vancomycin in a clinical setting. Since vancomycin is so powerful and its

25. See "Disease 'Crisis' Predicted" (1996); "Bacteria Repel Antibiotics in N.Y. Hospital Patients" (1996); "Incidence of Drug-Resistant Bacteria Soars since '94" (1997); and Gold and Moellering (1996).

26. "Drug-Resistant Germ Shows up in U.S." (1997); "Drug-Resistant Germ Found" (1997).

role as the last resort antibiotic is so important, attempts are being made to severely restrict its use to avoid bacteria developing resistance to it.[27] Such use restrictions may have significant effects on firms' incentives to develop new last resort antibiotics.[28]

In theory, the existence of these negative externalities might increase incentives for pharmaceutical manufacturers to innovate and develop new antibiotics. First, the existence of overprescription may allow manufacturers to keep prices higher than they would otherwise be, increasing profit margins for antibiotics. Second, the growing frequency of drug resistance should induce manufacturers to develop new antibiotics that are not susceptible to resistance. In practice, however, these incentives may not be high enough to induce firms to invest in large, sunk research and development costs.

It might appear, then, that the positive and negative externalities from the use of antibiotics counteract each other, making it difficult to draw conclusions about what the impact of these externalities is on innovation in antibiotics and whether innovation is too high or too low relative to what it should be. Indeed, the question of how externalities are affecting innovation has been the subject of many recent discussions.[29] What has been missed in all of these discussions, however, is one feature of resistance transmission that may actually serve to make the negative externality reinforce the impact of the positive externality, and that therefore may be important for thinking about incentives to innovate and develop new antibiotics.

One way to minimize the negative externality of resistance transmission is to rotate the use of different antibiotics in a particular clinical setting, such as a hospital, so that the bacteria cannot "learn" how to become resistant to any particular drug. If decisionmakers do not properly take into account resistance transmission, they will essentially undervalue the use of variety in the choice of antibiotics in treating bacterial infections. What does this imply about incentives to innovate and develop new antibiotics? More variety is brought about by more innovation, so if society undervalues variety, society will undervalue new antibiotics, meaning that the demand for new drugs will be lower than it

27. A recent report, however, states that CDC guidelines for vancomycin use are being violated routinely ("Wide Overuse of Antibiotic Cited in Study" [1997]).

28. At least two new antibiotics that show action against vancomycin-resistant strains are in the pipeline, however: Synercid by Rhone-Poulenc Rorer, which is currently under review for FDA approval; and Daptomycin by Eli Lilly and Company and Cubist Pharmaceuticals.

29. See U.S. Congress (1995) and the references therein.

should be. This is particularly true if newly developed antibiotics are more expensive than existing drugs and if people would prefer, all else equal, to pay less for drugs.[30] The negative externality of undervaluation of variety means that there is less incentive to innovate than there would be in the absence of externalities. So in this case, the negative externality of drug resistance, as captured by undervaluation of variety, actually reinforces the reduced incentives to innovate that are created by the positive externalities of antibiotics use.

To help clarify this idea, we develop in the appendix a simple mathematical model of antibiotics use in society where we incorporate the positive externalities of reduced disease transmission and the negative externalities of the undervaluation of variety in antibiotics use and examine the implications of these externalities on private market demand relative to the social optimum.

Ultimately, whether incentives to innovate are too low or too high relative to the social optimum will depend on a host of factors related to the positive and negative externalities. The magnitudes of these different factors are unknown and should be a key feature of future research. We note that an additional and no less important factor determining incentives to innovate is the magnitude of price competition in antibiotics. As we discuss above, our price indexes do not tell us anything directly about price competition in antibiotics, except to suggest that as consolidation in the delivery of health care continues and decisions about pharmaceutical prescriptions are made by agents with more and more bargaining power (such as hospitals and HMOs), there is likely to be less room for large markups in pharmaceuticals.

Conclusion

The price growth of antibiotics has been very modest over the last decade. Given the institutional history of antibiotics, this may not be surprising, although it is contrary to what government statistics suggest. It is worth noting that the evidence of modest price growth that we find comes solely from computations of traditional price indexes. Since consumers do not care about the intrinsic cost of a given health care treatment but about the cost of treating and curing diseases and maintaining

---

30. Alternatively, if the new drugs have other positive features that the private market does value, then private demand for new antibiotics will incorporate these positive features but will not fully incorporate the benefits of variety, so demand for the new antibiotic will be lower than it should be.

health, traditional antibiotics price indexes capture only part of the picture. If antibiotics are now being used as substitutes for costlier treatments, such as hospitalization, our traditional price indexes will understate the cost savings from using antibiotics to treat bacterial infections.[31]

Normally, low price growth is good news for consumers. There is, however, the potential for very bad news about antibiotics in the not-too-distant future. The growth of drug resistance is generally perceived as a problem for society, but the impact of the negative externality of drug resistance on society has not been fully understood. We present a simple model that illustrates how, contrary to intuition, the positive and negative externalities of antibiotics use may actually reinforce one another and reduce incentives to innovate and develop new drugs that may combat drug resistance. This feature of antibiotics use has been ignored in previous discussions about antibiotics and innovation.

We cannot argue that these factors establish that incentives to innovate in antibiotics are socially suboptimal. Rather, we argue that antibiotics deserve special treatment in discussions of the economics of pharmaceuticals, particularly incentives to innovate, because of their unique economic characteristics. These factors deserve more research and should be kept in mind during policy discussions of potential government involvement in the market for antibiotics, particularly with respect to discussions about public funding of R&D for new antibiotics.

The impact of recent increases in managed care on the structure of the antibiotics market is still unclear. It is likely that price competition will intensify as large managed care companies insist that pharmaceutical companies bid against one another for their business. The effect of the changes in health care on externalities in this market are more ambiguous. Cost containment may induce physicians to disregard externalities to the extent that physicians have to focus more on the private outcomes of patients in their practice. On the other hand, as health systems become more integrated, cost containment may lead to more emphasis on externalities, since effectively they will be internalized by the system. On the private side, cost-sensitive physicians may prescribe antibiotics less often when these prescriptions affect their bottom line, but to the extent that

31. For example, until recently, all very young children with high fevers were routinely hospitalized while awaiting test results to rule out potentially fatal bacterial infections. Only a very small percentage of those hospitalized children actually had a serious bacterial infection. Now, there is an antibiotic (ceftriaxone) that can be given in an outpatient setting to these children while awaiting the test results. The cost savings from eliminating these "rule-out" hospitalizations may be very important in reducing the costs of treating fever in children, but these cost savings are not captured in traditional price indexes, which would solely measure the price growth of ceftriaxone over time.

prescriptions may be a substitute for costlier treatment, such as an office consultation, antibiotics prescriptions could increase.

Appendix: A Model of the Externalities of Antibiotics Use

In the following case of one antibiotic, we examine the countervailing forces of the positive and negative externalities in the simplest setting imaginable. We learn from this case just what ordinary intuition tells us: positive and negative externalities have opposite and offsetting effects on demand, and parameters of the model—how easily resistance is spread, discount factors, and so on—will determine which effect prevails. We offer this case to establish notation and modeling strategy, to make the trade-offs of use of the antibiotic explicit, and to serve as a counterpoint to our results from the case of two antibiotics, by far the more interesting case. In the case of two antibiotics we show the vital importance of introducing variety into the model and find the counterintuitive result that the positive and negative externalities of antibiotics use may actually reinforce rather than cancel out one another.

We have obviously simplified the setting for antibiotics use for model ing purposes, leaving out many important features. We abstract away from a number of the issues critical to the question of innovation in antibiotics, including broad versus narrow spectrum antibiotics, the de- velopment of vaccines for use in prevention of bacterial infections, and use of practices that either encourage or inhibit resistance for a given level of antibiotics use.[32] As mentioned elsewhere in this chapter, we have chosen to do this because although the interaction between the externalities that our model illustrates has not been previously devel- oped, the other issues related to externalities have been explored.[33] Fi- nally, we have simplified the model itself in many ways in order to ensure tractability and ease of explication, but none of these simplifications (including the two-period, nonoverlapping nature of the model and the functional form assumptions) affects the important intuition.

The Case of One Antibiotic

Consider a two-period world with a population of N individuals who live in period $t = 1$ (and die at the end of the period) and an equally sized population of N individuals who live in period $t = 2$. People are either

---

32. We do return to a brief discussion of these other issues later.
33. For a comprehensive review, see U.S. Congress (1995).

sick or healthy, and this is known before the consumption decision. All people are endowed with income Y.[34] There is a consumption good C with price equal to 1, and one antibiotic with price p. There is no discount rate between the two periods.

When a person alive in period 1 is sick, his utility is defined as

$$(4\text{-}1) \qquad\qquad U(C_1, a_1) = a_1\left(\alpha + \frac{1}{2}\beta C_1\right),$$

where a_1 is the level of antibiotic used by the individual and C_1 is his consumption. Note that if the individual uses no antibiotic, utility is 0. The individual alive in period 1 has a budget constraint of

$$(4\text{-}2) \qquad\qquad Y = C_1 + p a_1.$$

For simplicity, assume that in period $t = 1$, all people are sick. The level of antibiotic use, a_1^*, that maximizes utility for each of these N people subject to their budget constraint is:

$$(4\text{-}3) \qquad\qquad a_{1_p}^* = \frac{\alpha + \frac{1}{2}\beta Y}{\beta p}.$$

The addition of the subscript p in equation (4-3) denotes that this is the private (not social) optimal level of antibiotics consumption for period 1 individuals.

In period $t = 2$, however, the probability that an individual is sick is e^{-Na_1}, a decreasing function of the amount of antibiotic used by each individual in the first period.[35] This term reflects the positive externality of antibiotic use—when an individual used the antibiotic in period 1, the probability that a person in period 2 will be sick goes down.

Conditional on a person's being sick in period 2, his or her utility function is slightly different than for a period 1 individual:

$$(4\text{-}4) \qquad\qquad U(C_2, a_2 \mid S_2) = \frac{a_2}{e^{rNa_1}}\left(\alpha + \frac{1}{2}\beta C_2\right).$$

---

34. Incomes could differ between the two periods without affecting the results.

35. Since all individuals in period 1 are sick and otherwise identical, they will all choose to consume the same amount of antibiotic.

The extra term in the utility function of sick people in period 2, e^{-rNa_1}, is the "resistance effect." This term can be thought of as reflecting the diminished effectiveness of period 2 antibiotic use that comes with drug resistance. Here, r is a constant representing the degree to which extra antibiotic use creates resistance. As the amount of period 1 use of the antibiotic increases, the effectiveness of period 2 antibiotic use, a_2, goes down and utility decreases as a result. This is the negative externality associated with use of the antibiotic.[36]

The probability that a period 2 person will be healthy is $(1 - e^{-Na_1})$, and conditional on being healthy, a person's utility function is

$$(4\text{-}5) \qquad U(C_2, a_2 | H_2) = \alpha + \frac{1}{2}\beta C_2.$$

So a healthy person in period 2 will not consume any antibiotic.

To summarize, higher period 1 antibiotic use causes lower incidence of illness in period 2, but those illnesses are more serious, require more treatment, and lower utility of those who are sick.

The world ends after period 2. Period 2 individuals, therefore, create no externalities.

Assume now that there is a social planner whose objective function maximizes the sum of individuals' utilities across both periods. The social planner cannot reallocate income across individuals but can determine optimal consumption and antibiotic use for each individual. So the social planner's objective function is

$$(4\text{-}6) \qquad \begin{aligned} \max_{a_1, a_2} \ & Na_1 \left(\alpha + \frac{1}{2}\beta(Y - pa_1) \right) \\ & + Ne^{-Na_1} \frac{a_2}{e^{rNa_1}} \left[\alpha + \frac{1}{2}\beta(Y - pa_2) \right] \\ & + N(1 - e^{-Na_1}) \left(\alpha + \frac{1}{2}\beta Y \right). \end{aligned}$$

Since period 2 individuals create no externalities, the private optimum that period 2 individuals will choose is equivalent to the social planner's

---

36. One could augment the model to allow for the possibility of death prior to consumption, where the probability of death would increase with drug resistance. This is done in Garber (1982), where antibiotics are assumed to be costless. Here, adding in death as an outcome does not change the signs of the results of the model, but the fact that there is a cost to antibiotic use in this model makes it difficult to incorporate death and still obtain closed form solutions.

optimum. Period 2 decisions about consumption and antibiotic use can then be left aside, and the decision variable of interest becomes antibiotic use in period 1. Since individuals are identical, the social planner can solve the problem by choosing the optimal antibiotic use for any one individual. The first order condition for the socially optimal level of antibiotic use for each person in period 1 is the a_{1s}^* that solves

(4-7)
$$\alpha + \frac{1}{2}\beta Y - \beta p a_{1s}^* - N(1+r)e^{-N(1+r)a_{1s}^*}$$
$$\left[a_2 \left(\alpha + \frac{1}{2}\beta(Y - pa_2) \right) \right] + Ne^{-Na_{1s}^*}\left(\alpha + \frac{1}{2}\beta Y \right) = 0.$$

Rearranging the first order condition in equation (4-7) yields:

(4-8)
$$\frac{\alpha + \frac{1}{2}\beta Y}{\beta p} = a_{1s}^* + \left(\frac{1}{\beta p} \right) Ne^{-Na_{1s}^*}$$
$$\left[(1+r)e^{-rNa_{1s}^*}\left(a_2\left(\alpha + \frac{1}{2}\beta(Y - pa_2) \right) \right) - \left(\alpha + \frac{1}{2}\beta Y \right) \right].$$

Note that the term on the left side of equation (4-8) is the private optimum, a_{1p}^*. Whether the social optimum, a_{1s}^*, will be smaller or larger than the private optimum depends on the relative magnitudes of the two terms inside square brackets. Both terms are positive, and the second, $\left(\alpha + \frac{1}{2}\beta Y \right)$, is subtracted from the first, $(1+r)e^{-rNa_{1s}^*}$ $\left(a_2\left(\alpha + \frac{1}{2}\beta(Y - pa_2) \right) \right)$. Note that the second term is the utility of a healthy person in period 2, and the first term is $(1 + r)$ times the utility of a sick person in period 2.

If the first term is bigger than the second term, $a_{1s}^* < a_{1p}^*$, this may be interpreted as saying that the relative importance to society of reducing resistance in the second period is greater than that of reducing illness, so the social optimum is below the private optimum. More people will be sick under the social optimum than under the private optimum in this case, but their utility gain from reduced resistance will more than make up for the extra sickness. Conversely, if the second term in the equation is bigger than the first term, then $a_{1s}^* > a_{1p}^*$. In this case, it is relatively more important to keep people healthy than to keep sick people from suffering a utility loss from drug resistance.

This very simple case is valuable to establish the trade-off between the positive externality (reduced transmission of illness) and the negative externality (increased drug resistance) of antibiotic use. Whether actual antibiotic use in this model is higher or lower than the social optimum is determined by the constant, r, representing the degree to which extra antibiotic use creates resistance. It is clear that for some values of r, those for which resistance is less easily created, demand for the antibiotic will be lower than is socially optimal. Although we do not explicitly model firms' decisions in this context, it is clear that lower than optimal demand would mean lower incentives for firms to incur the costs necessary to bring other antibiotics to market relative to their incentives in the absence of externalities.

In the context of this very simple case, higher values of r would imply the opposite result: demand higher than optimal, leading to higher incentives for firms to innovate. This model, however, abstracts away from a very important feature of the market for antibiotics—variety. Recall that variety and the ability to rotate antibiotics can be effective in decreasing resistance for a given level of antibiotics use. We will see that when we enrich the model to include variety, our result can imply that the negative externality of resistance transmission can actually reinforce the positive externality in lowering incentives to innovate.

The Case of Two Antibiotics

Assume now that there are two antibiotics in the world as otherwise described above, one selling at price p_e and one at price p_n, where $p_e > p_n$. One can think of the expensive antibiotic as a new antibiotic that has just appeared on the market. Both antibiotics are equally effective at reducing illness and increasing utility. The only difference between the two antibiotics from an individual's point of view is the price difference between them. Moreover, the rate of sickness transmission between periods 1 and 2 is a function of the total use of antibiotics by period 1 individuals. There is a difference, however, in how resistance is transmitted between the two periods: now, the "resistance effect," r, in the utility function of a sick person in period 2 is not a constant but rather a function of the ratios in which the two drugs are used by society. This means that there is an optimal mix of the two drugs to be used in the first period.

Sick individuals only use one type of antibiotic. Let A_{1n} be the total amount of the inexpensive antibiotic used in the first period, and let A_{1e} be the total amount of the expensive antibiotic used in the first period. Then define A_1, overall antibiotics use in the first period, to be $A_1 = A_{1n} + A_{1e}$.

Let the resistance effect r be

$$(4\text{-}9) \qquad r = \frac{\left(A_{1n} - \frac{1}{2}A_1\right)\left(\frac{1}{2}A_1 - A_{1e}\right)}{A_1},$$

or

$$(4\text{-}10) \qquad r = \frac{\left(A_{1n} - \frac{1}{2}A_1\right)^2}{A_1^2}.$$

Then conditional on being sick, an individual in period 2 has utility function

$$(4\text{-}11) \qquad U\left(C_2, a_2 | S_2\right) = e^{\frac{-\left(A_{1n} - \frac{1}{2}A_1\right)^2}{A_1}} a_2\left(\alpha + \frac{1}{2}\beta(Y - P_n a_2)\right).$$

Note that since sick people in period 2 create no externalities, they will use the inexpensive antibiotic under both the private and the social optimum. The utility functions of all other individuals are the same as in the previous section, and total income and the price of consumption are unchanged.

Obviously, in the case of the private optimum, period 1 individuals will all choose the inexpensive antibiotic, since the only difference to them between the two antibiotics is the price. It is easy to see that having only one type of antibiotic used in period 1 will maximize the level of r in period 2 (conditional on the total amount of antibiotics used.)

To examine the case of the optimal mix of drugs under the social planner's problem, assume that the level of total antibiotics consumed in period 1, A_1, is fixed. This allows us to focus solely on the optimal mix of the two existing antibiotics.

The social planner has to choose both the overall level of each type of antibiotic to be consumed (which amounts to choosing A_{1n}, since A_1 is fixed) and the number of sick individuals $N_n \leq N$ in period 1 over which to divide A_1.[37]

The social planner's problem can therefore be written as

(4-12)
$$
\begin{aligned}
\max_{N_n, A_{1n}} \; & A_{1n}\left[\alpha + \frac{1}{2}\beta\left(Y - p_n \frac{A_{1n}}{N_n}\right)\right] \\
& + A_{1e}\left[\alpha + \frac{1}{2}\beta\left(Y - p_e \frac{A_{1e}}{N - N_n}\right)\right] \\
& + Ne^{-A_1}e^{\frac{-\left(A_{1n} - \frac{1}{2}A_1\right)^2}{A_1}} a_2\left[\alpha + \frac{1}{2}\beta(Y - p_n a_2)\right] \\
& + N\left(1 - e^{-A_1}\right)\left[\alpha + \frac{1}{2}\beta Y\right].
\end{aligned}
$$

There are two first order conditions, one for A_{1n}, and one for N_n. The equations are complicated, but after manipulating them and substituting the first order condition for N_n into the first order condition for A_{1n}, one can obtain the following equation:

(4-13)
$$
\begin{aligned}
& \beta\sqrt{p_n}\sqrt{p_n}\left(\frac{A_1 - A_{1n}}{N - N_n}\right) + \beta p_e\left(\frac{A_{1n} - A_1}{N - N_n}\right) \\
& + 2N\left(\frac{A_{1n} - \frac{1}{2}A_1}{A_1}\right)e^{-A_1}e^{\frac{-\left(A_{1n} - \frac{1}{2}A_1\right)^2}{A_1}} a_2\left[\alpha + \frac{1}{2}\beta(Y - p_n a_2)\right] = 0.
\end{aligned}
$$

The first term in equation (4-13) is nonnegative (as long as both antibiotics are consumed in period 1), while the second term is nonpositive. Notice, however, that as long as $A_{1n} < A_1$, the second term is larger than the first in absolute value since $p_e > p_n$. Moreover, it has to be the case that $A_{1n} < A_1$ in order for the equality in equation (4-13) to hold. Therefore, the sum of the first two terms is negative, which means that the third term must be positive. Therefore, the optimal level of A_{1n} is greater than $\frac{1}{2}A_1$, but less than A_1.

---

37. Note that this is equivalent to choosing N_n and the level of inexpensive antibiotics consumed by each of these individuals, a_n.

Note that if $p_n = p_e$ so that the drugs are equally priced, then the optimal mix of antibiotics between the expensive and inexpensive drugs splits A_1 equally between them. This makes sense, since if the drugs are equally priced, individuals in period 1 will be indifferent between the two drugs, so conditional on the overall level of antibiotics consumed in the first period, the social planner will want to minimize resistance. This occurs when $A_{1n} = A_{1e} = \frac{1}{2}A_1$. If, however, one drug is less expensive, the social planner will choose to allocate more than half of period 1 consumption to that drug, but it will still be optimal to have some consumption of the more expensive drug in the first period to help lower resistance.

What does this all imply about innovation of new antibiotics? The intuition is straightforward. New innovation brings variety, which, as we noted above, has been found to help combat resistance. But if newly developed drugs are more expensive than existing drugs, the private market will not demand them, so the private market again provides less incentive to innovate than it would in the absence of externalities.[38]

References

"Bacteria Repel Antibiotics in N.Y. Hospital Patients." 1996. *USA Today* (November 22).

Baye, Michael, Robert Maness, and Steven Wiggins. 1992. "Demand Systems and the 'True' Subindex of the Cost-of-Living for Pharmaceuticals." Department of Economics, Texas A&M University.

Berndt, Ernst R., Zvi Griliches, and Joshua G. Rosett. 1993. "Auditing the Producer Price Index: Micro Evidence from Prescription Pharmaceutical Products." *Journal of Business and Economic Statistics* 11(3): 251–64.

BLS Handbook of Methods. 1997. U.S. Department of Labor, Bureau of Labor Statistics.

Boston Consulting Group. 1993. "The Changing Environment for U.S. Pharmaceuticals." Mimeo. Boston.

"Disease 'Crisis' Predicted." 1996. *Boston Globe* (May 20).

Drug Facts and Comparisons. 1991. St. Louis: Lippincott.

"Drug Makers Go All out to Squash 'Superbugs.'" 1996. *Wall Street Journal* (June 25).

"Drug-Resistant Germ Found." 1997. *New York Times* (September 5).

"Drug-Resistant Germ Shows up in U.S." 1997. *New York Times* (August 22).

Ellison, Sara Fisher, and others. 1997. "Characteristics of Demand for Pharmaceutical Products: An Examination of Four Cephalosporins." *RAND Journal of Economics* 28 (3):426–46.

---

38. Or, if new drugs have other positive features that are valued by the private market, then private demand will be too low.

Frank, R., and E. Berndt. 1997. "Prices for Treatment of Depression." National Bureau of Economic Research.

Garber, Alan. 1982. "Cost and Control of Antibiotic Resistance." Ph.D. dissertation, Harvard University.

Gold, Howard S., and Robert C. Moellering Jr. 1996. "Drug Therapy: Antimicrobial Drug Resistance." *New England Journal of Medicine* 355:1445–52.

Griliches, Zvi, and Iain Cockburn. 1994. "Generics and New Goods in Pharmaceutical Price Indexes." *American Economic Review* 4(5): 1213–32.

Hellerstein, Judith K. 1995. "Economic Impediments to the Development of New Antibiotic Drugs." Office of Technology Assessment, U.S. Congress.

———. 1998. "The Importance of the Physician in the Generic versus Trade-Name Prescription Decision." *RAND Journal of Economics* 29(10): 108—36.

"Incidence of Drug-Resistant Bacteria Soars since '94." 1997. *USA Today* (April 19).

Kanoza, Douglas. 1996. "Supplemental Sampling in the PPI Pharmaceuticals Index." Bureau of Labor Statistics. *PPI Detailed Report,* 8–10.

Newhouse, Joseph P., and the Insurance Experiment Group. 1993. *Free for All? Lessons from the Rand Health Insurance Experiment.* Harvard University Press.

Physicians Desk Reference. 1993. New York: Medical Economics Data.

"A Shift of Power in Pharmaceuticals." 1994. *New York Times* (May 9).

Tomasz, Alexander. 1994. "Multiple-Antibiotic-Resistant Pathogenic Bacteria." *New England Journal of Medicine* 330: 1247–51.

U.S. Congress, Office of Technology Assessment. 1995. "Impacts of Antibiotic-Resistant Bacteria." OTA-H-629. Washington, D.C.

"Wide Overuse of Antibiotic Cited in Study." 1997. *Wall Street Journal* (September 4).

Wiggins, Steven, and Robert Maness. 1995. "Price Competition in Pharmaceuticals: The Case of Antiinfectives." Department of Economics, Texas A&M University.

Comments on
Chapter 4

COMMENT BY

Thomas W. Croghan

CHAPTER 4 DEALS with difficult issues regarding the incentives that affect pharmaceutical company decisions to invest in discovery research and development. The Ellison and Hellerstein study suggests that marketplace forces, specifically competition that limits price growth and hence firms' ability to recoup research and development costs, have resulted in suboptimal innovation of new antibiotics.

The authors address the issue of pharmaceutical innovation from two perspectives. First, they propose a theoretical model to account for externalities imposed by the fact that antibiotic use by an individual has effects on others. An empirical model of pricing of one class of antibiotics, the cephalosporins, is presented to account for other issues related to innovation.

The theoretical model of antibiotics use results in the conclusion that the positive externality created by limiting the spread of infectious disease and the negative externality created by increased resistance to antibiotics both result in reductions in the incentive to innovate. At least one of these findings seems counterintuitive. Although it makes sense that reduced demand would result in less incentive to create new antibiotics, creating resistant strains of bacteria seems likely to increase demand for new antibiotics and thus incentives to innovate. Even though there is a lag between initial creation of resistant strains and widespread need for a new antibiotic, the pharmaceutical industry has historically taken a risk on perceived medical need and seems likely to attempt to meet the need.

There is thus a gap between the implications of the theoretical model and the intuitive that must be explained. There are two assumptions of the models that seem likely to bridge this gap. First, the concept of two sequential and nonoverlapping time periods is of concern. It results in the conclusion that antibiotic use in the first period results in fewer sick individuals in the second. This assumption may or may not hold true. It seems much more likely that antibiotic use in period 1 would reduce the incidence and prevalence of the infection in period 1 and that incidence in period 2 would be only marginally affected by period 1 use. For example, the incidence of pneumonia in any particular year is much more dependent on the incidence and severity of the prevailing strain of influenza than on antibiotic use in the prior flu season. This notion lends itself to the concept of an overlapping generations model, a potentially formidable task, but such an effort would result in a model that would fit clinical experience.

Second, the model ignores the current reality of multiple antibiotics that are used to treat many different illnesses and that may share one or more resistance mechanisms. When multiple antibiotics are available, infection control models generally follow a sequential pathway whereby one antibiotic, usually the most expensive, is reserved for circumstances when resistance has been demonstrated in a particular institution. In other words, there is variety of use, but often the variety occurs within a class of antibiotics, or through use of drugs with the same primary resistance mechanism.

The empirical evidence of antibiotic pricing is interesting and important in its own right. The pharmaceutical industry has been the subject of intense pricing pressure, at least in part because of the impression that prices have been rising faster than general inflation, even though recent evidence suggests otherwise.[1] The findings regarding distribution channels also seem sensible. The move toward ambulatory care as an expense control has made hospital markets less important to pharmaceutical companies. Furthermore, managed care companies have recognized the value of substituting pharmaceuticals for other services, so they appear to demand more drugs, with resulting increase in prices.

The more important aspects of both the theoretical model and the empirical data relate to the apparent failure of current incentives to provide an adequate incentive for innovation in what appears to be a crisis in the making. And a crisis it could be. At Lilly, we estimated a few years ago that widespread resistance to the common treatments for ear infections in children would add about $20 billion to current U.S. health care expendi-

1. Berndt, Cockburn, and Griliches (1996).

tures.[2] Comments on how pharmaceutical companies make investment decisions may add to the discussion. As a first approximation, pharmaceutical companies base research and development decisions on four dimensions: medical need, resources and development time required, technical feasibility, and market potential. Of these, chapter 4 relates mostly to the medical need and market potential dimensions. Assessment of medical need is based on both the incidence or prevalence of the condition and the severity of its impact on an individual. The question is posed to scientific and medical staff and advisors and in many cases is not assessed by marketing departments. So one might imagine that considerations of resistance and spread of disease would be viewed from the societal perspective, and indeed they are. But in contrast to other conditions, such as mental illness, the perceived medical need for new, broad spectrum antibiotics is relatively low. Scientists would rather concentrate on the specific but difficult problems of antibiotic resistance mechanisms.

The market potential is determined by a mix of objective and subjective considerations on the part of marketing departments regarding potential price and volume. From the perspective of a marketing department, the worldwide antibiotics market is very large, and therefore almost any new entry has some potential for profitability. Expansion into new markets seems unlikely. In years past, the way to gain market share was to produce an antibiotic that met multiple needs; in others words, an antibiotic with a broader spectrum. But we seem to have approached an optimum from this strategy, and I suggest that the Ellison-Hellerstein model, and their empirical study of the current markets, predicts this aspect of pharmaceutical investment quite well. The fact that we do not seem to need new broad spectrum antibiotics does not, however, dissuade companies from support for new and more specific antibiotics.

COMMENT BY
Patricia M. Danzon

CHAPTER 4 ADDRESSES the discrepancy between the privately optimal use and the socially optimal use of antibiotics, with potentially important implications for research and development incentives. This discrepancy can arise from two factors: the positive externality of reduced disease transmission, and the negative

2. Croghan (1994).

externality of increasing bacterial resistance, which reduces the efficacy of drugs in future treatment.

The challenge in analyzing this complex problem is whether theoretical modeling yields insights that are plausible and go beyond those provided by simple intuition. In the simple model with a single drug, the conclusion is that the private optimum may be too high or too low, depending on whether the "relative importance of reducing resistance is greater than that of reducing illness." This is true but was known at the outset so this formulation adds little new. The model becomes more interesting when multiple drugs are included. This seems to tip the balance toward suboptimal private use. In the Ellison-Hellerstein model, innovation is much more likely to be too low because private demand fails not only to reflect the positive social value of reducing contagion but also to internalize the value of varying use in order to reduce resistance.

However, this conclusion, that private demand for new drugs and hence research and development is likely to be too low once we take into account drug variety, depends critically on the assumption that both drugs have the same effect on resistance. In this model, resistance is unidimensional (there is only one type of bacterium) and depends only on total antibiotic use and the variance in total use.

In fact, dynamic competition in antibiotic research and development takes the form of introducing broader spectrum compounds that attack a wider range of bacteria and hence are more likely to be effective. But this characteristic that makes new drugs more effective, and hence have higher private value, also induces broader resistance, and hence has a greater negative externality. If this assumption is correct, that the characteristic that makes new antibiotics more effective also entails higher resistance costs, then it is not obvious that private demand for new drugs is suboptimal relative to their private efficacy, nor is it clear that the rate of innovation is suboptimal. Indeed, if individuals are risk averse, it is quite possible that the private incentive is to use a broad spectrum drug when a narrower spectrum one would probably do the job, and hence that firms face incentives to broaden the spectrum of new drugs too rapidly. In fact both outcomes may be possible—that is, market forces may create incentives for too few new drugs but with an excessively broad spectrum of action that yields a socially excessive spread of resistance. Thus with this changed and, I believe, more realistic assumption about the nature of innovation, the conclusions from the formal model are still ambiguous.

Of course, if the intent is to draw practical policy conclusions about tax subsidies and so forth, then the usual and more complete list of distortions in medical markets must be taken into account. Even if the net effect—sign and magnitude—of externalities from antibiotic use could be determined by modifying the current model, distortions not addressed in this chapter due to such factors as insurance-induced moral hazard, imperfect information, and agency on the part of physicians should be considered before voting for policy action.

The empirical analysis does not directly address the discrepancy between private incentives and the socially optimal use of antibiotics, which admittedly would not be easy to do. Rather, the authors calculate indexes of price change for the cephalosporin class. Finding that the real rate of price increase over time has been low or negative, they conclude that this market is highly competitive, which would tend to reinforce the disincentive for innovation.

However, this index for the cephalosporin class in aggregate suppresses detail on quality improvement over time, due to entry of second and third generation products and changes in dosage forms, pack sizes, strengths, and so on. To examine incentives for innovation, it would be more instructive to disaggregate the data to compare relative prices and volumes of new drugs and to old drugs. The casual evidence is that new products are priced at a significant multiple relative to old drugs, and volume at these high relative prices is far from zero, contrary to the predictions of the authors' model. The evidence from the disaggregated data would almost certainly show stronger incentives for innovation than are suggested by the aggregate price indexes presented, although conclusions about whether incentives for innovation are too high or too low would still remain indeterminate. More generally, even if one could observe the relation between price and marginal cost, this conveys little information about overall profitability because over 50 percent of total costs for research-based pharmaceuticals are fixed costs of research and development, production capacity, and other overhead.

A further problem is that the reported data from IMS do not accurately measure prices to manufacturers. These data are based on wholesale invoices, which do not reflect rebates and other discounts that are paid directly to final purchasers. The frequency of such discounts has almost certainly increased over time, with the growth of managed pharmacy benefits, but trends in the average magnitude of discounts are not known. It seems likely that the increased frequency effect dominates, hence that these price indexes based on wholesale prices overstate the growth in manufacturer net revenues over time.

The more rapid rate of increase for HMOs than for hospitals is puzzling. The authors attribute this to the decline in discounts given to HMOs, presumably due to the Medicaid "best price" provision, which, since 1990, requires companies to give the lowest price offered to any private purchaser to Medicaid and other public payers. However, to the extent that wholesale price data here are gross of discounts, they would not reflect changes in discounts; moreover, any incentive for manufacturers to reduce discounts due to the best price law would apply to hospitals as well as to HMOs.

Two other possible explanations are worth considering, in addition to those mentioned by Tom Croghan. First, it is possible that HMOs have shifted more to newer, higher-priced products within the class, whereas hospitals have continued to use relatively more of the older, cheaper, narrower spectrum products. This would be consistent with the hypothesis that hospitals have stronger incentives to internalize the negative externality of excessive use of broad spectrum products that generate broader resistance. Unfortunately, there are also other plausible explanations, such as different market incentives. Specifically, HMOs may respond to their need to compete for patients and physicians directly by offering the most effective drugs available. Second but related, the HMO series may also be biased by change in the mix of HMOs that operate their own pharmacies, to include more group and IPA models that may offer a broader formulary than the staff model HMOs that were the first to operate their own pharmacies.

COMMENT BY
Henry Grabowski

B OTH CHAPTERS 4 and 5 are interesting and provocative. Together they consider an array of potential market failures or incentive problems relevant to the drug innovation process. They show that there are many situations that can lead to an underproduction of knowledge with respect to new and established drug therapies. They also set forth a menu of policy options for dealing with these market failures.

Ellison and Hellerstein focus on one particular class of drug therapies, namely, antibiotics. Their main contribution is a rigorous modeling framework to consider the externality conditions that can lead to inadequate investment incentives for new antibiotics. There are also some related empirical analyses of antibiotic prices, but the heart of the chapter appears to be its theoretical study of externality effects on innovation incentives.

The main insight gained from Ellison and Hellerstein's model is that the positive externality from consuming antibiotics (from the reduced transmission of illness) reinforces the negative externality (from increased drug resistance). Together they decrease the incentives for antibiotic innovation below optimal levels. This is not an intuitively obvious result. Their two-period model is constructed to show how price competition between new and older antibiotic drugs is a key factor underlying this finding. Of course, as the authors recognize, their model necessarily abstracts from a number of factors. In addition, as Professor Danzon's comments indicate, it remains to be seen whether their model is robust to alternative specifications.

One important factor that the Ellison-Hellerstein model does not consider is the possibility of alternative medical options. For example, many of the bacterial infections that can be treated by antibiotics could in principle be prevented by vaccines. Vaccines share some of the same characteristics as antibiotics (the positive externality from reduced disease transmission), but not others (the possibility of drug resistance). All theoretical models in economics necessarily abstract from many relevant factors in order to be tractable. Nevertheless, if the Ellison-Hellerstein model is to be utilized as the basis for policy actions (such as targeted tax subsidies and government grants), it is clearly essential to consider additional factors, such as the role of alternative medical options.

Economic studies have shown very high social benefit-cost ratios for most of our current pediatric vaccines—the measles, mumps, and rubella vaccine; the diphtheria, pertussis, and tetanus vaccine; the oral polio vaccine; and so forth. Nevertheless, research and development expenditures for new vaccines have historically been dwarfed by research and development expenditures on new antibiotics. The incentives for vaccine research and development have been adversely affected by several factors, including (1) a health care insurance system that has traditionally favored treatment over prevention; (2) extra regulatory hurdles for vaccines because they are biologicals; (3) higher liability risks for vaccines; and (4) the presence of the government as a major purchaser of vaccines at below market prices. These factors caused most of the pharmaceutical firms to exit the vaccine business in the 1970s and 1980s.[3] By the mid-

3. Institute of Medicine (1985).

1980s, only three domestic drug firms were still manufacturing pediatric vaccines.

It is worth noting that over the last decade there has been a renaissance in vaccine innovation. New vaccines are in development for many bacterial and viral infections such as Lyme disease, tuberculosis, malaria, otitis media, and herpes.[4] This renewed research and development activity has been fostered by new opportunities for vaccines through advances in biotechnology and related scientific fields. Several biotech firms have entered into the discovery research phase for vaccines. Many of the factors holding back vaccine research and development have also turned around in the last decade. But there also remain large uncertainties concerning public policies toward vaccine purchases at the present time.[5]

In terms of the Ellison-Hellerstein analysis of antibiotics, vaccines are an alternative, but sometimes complementary, approach to disease eradication. They clearly play an important role in the determination of whether the research and development incentives for antibiotics are suboptimal. They also influence the appropriate policy prescriptions in particular disease categories. The interactions between preventive and treatment approaches to infectious diseases remain an important issue for further research.

References

Berndt, Ernst R., Iaian Cockburn, and Zvi Griliches. 1996. "Pharmaceutical Innovations and Market Dynamics: Tracking Effects on Price Indexes for Anti-Depressant Drugs." In *Brookings Papers: Microeconomics,* pp. 133-88.
Croghan, Thomas W. 1994. "Economics of Antibiotic Resistance." Technical report. Eli Lilly and Company.
Division of Microbiology and Infectious Diseases, National Institute of Allergy and Infectious Diseases. 1996. *The Jordan Report: Accelerated Development of Vaccines: Annual Report.* Bethesda, Md.: National Institutes of Health.
Grabowski, Henry, and John Vernon. 1997. *The Search for New Vaccines: The Effects of the Vaccines for Children Program.* Washington, D.C.: AEI Press.
Institute of Medicine. 1985. *Vaccine Supply and Innovation.* Washington, D.C.: National Academy Press.

4. Division of Microbiology and Infectious Diseases (1996).
5. Grabowski and Vernon (1997).

5

Drug Patents and Prices: Can We Achieve Better Outcomes?

Joel W. Hay and Winnie M. Yu

A CRUCIAL ISSUE in price index theory involves methods for appropriate adjustment of the prices in representative consumer market baskets when older products are supplanted by newer ones. A new product may have different characteristics, enhanced capabilities, or altered features that must be accounted for in determining how much of the expenditure change is due to pure price change and quality or quantity changes. This is particularly germane to pharmaceutical price indexes, since valuable new therapies are constantly being introduced to the marketplace, some representing superior therapies within an existing therapeutic class, others representing entirely novel treatments (for example, in recent years, the introduction of protease inhibitors to treat HIV infection). In a competitive market with perfect knowledge, if a new drug costs more than the drug it is replacing, it must have some additional clinical advantages (cures patients faster, uses fewer hospital resources, has a broader spectrum of activity, and so on).

Suppose the cost of the representative market basket of pharmaceuticals has increased when a new therapy replaces an old therapy. This could mean that prices have gone up while "outputs" (patient quality-adjusted outcomes) have stayed constant, that prices have stayed constant and "outputs" have increased, or an infinite number of combinations of drug price and drug output combinations. Meaningful policy evaluation of drug expenditures requires accurate measurement of the outcomes of

We thank Kevin Livengood, Rita Hui, Saresh Danani, Robert Ward, Jerry Avorn, Steve Finder, Brian Garofalo, Bill Comanor, and AEI/Brookings conference participants for their helpful comments.

drug therapies. Although the pharmaceutical marketplace has been quite successful in encouraging the development of new products, it has not been as successful in encouraging comprehensive drug outcome evaluation.

Over the past several decades, the U.S. pharmaceutical and biotechnology industry, in addition to representing one of the stronger success stories in recent national economic growth, has discovered and brought to market hundreds of important new products that have improved the health, survival, and well-being of people around the world. This has been accomplished in a government-regulated capitalist marketplace, with profit seeking by individual entrepreneurs and corporate shareholders as the primary motivator for success.

U.S. pharmaceutical companies account for 36 percent of global research and development spending (Japan 19 percent, Germany 10 percent, France 9 percent, and the United Kingdom 7 percent).[1] In sharp contrast to other industries, the U.S. pharmaceutical industry invests nearly a fifth of sales on research and development. For example, U.S. research-based pharmaceutical companies have over 300 cancer drugs in development and expect to invest more than $1.5 billion in cancer research this year alone.[2]

Pharmaceutical prices diverge from perfect competition, in large part because of patent protection. Patent protection and marketing exclusivity for new products is vital to pharmaceutical research and development. The cost of developing a single new drug rose from $54 million in 1976 to $359 million in 1990.[3] The average time required to bring a new drug through the FDA approval process has risen from 8.1 years in the 1960s to 14.8 years today (approximately two years slower than in the United Kingdom and other European countries), and generic competition has more than doubled in the past decade. A 1994 study by the Congressional Budget Office found that pharmaceutical company profits are about average for companies in all industries, despite the enormous risk associated with the drug discovery process.[4] Only 1 in 5,000 tested compounds makes it as an approved, marketed drug.[5]

1. Pharmaceutical Research and Manufacturers of America (1997).
2. Pharmaceutical Research and Manufacturers of America (1996), based on data from the PhRMA Annual Survey and data from Compustat, as published in "R&D Scoreboard," *Business Week* (July 1995).
3. DiMasi and others (1995), 152.
4. U.S. Congress, Office of Technology Assessment (1993).
5. Pharmaceutical Research and Manufacturers of America (1997).

The justification for patent protection is firmly established in theory and law. According to economic theory, unless innovators are allowed to capture a substantial portion of the gains of their innovative products through temporary monopoly protection (marketing exclusivity), the level of provision of innovative products will be substantially below that which would optimally benefit society. This is a classic public goods problem.[6] In an unregulated pharmaceutical market, if an innovator drug company were to invest millions of dollars in developing a new product without assurances of marketing exclusivity, a substantial portion of benefits of its investment would go to its competitors. The optimal pharmaceutical investment strategy would be to free-ride on the innovations of others. Important medicines with very high social rates of return on investment would remain undeveloped or be developed too slowly, and we would all be worse off.[7]

The current drug patent protection scheme, which generally provides an innovative drug with a minimum of five and a maximum of twenty years of marketing exclusivity after FDA marketing approval, is a trade-off between competing societal objectives. If there were perfect knowledge and zero transactions costs, the ideal patent protection scheme would be to reward the innovator with a lump sum payment reflecting the present discounted value of all consumer surpluses associated with demand for the medication and simultaneously to allow anyone to use or sell the medication from the time of marketing approval at marginal cost of production. Existing patent law recognizes that (1) the transactions costs associated with identification and extraction of consumer surplus are excessive, (2) absent perfect knowledge, manufacturers and consumers have strong incentives to misrepresent the value of a drug innovation, (3) absent perfect knowledge, large postmarket launch investments are often needed to educate providers and patients about the value of new pharmaceuticals, and (4) monopoly pricing with a fixed period of market exclusivity, although highly imprecise in addressing all these problems, provides a better societal outcome than an unregulated market.

Does current policy for patent protection and monopoly pricing of innovative medications achieve the best possible outcomes for society? We will argue that the answer is emphatically negative, for reasons that are unique to health care. Current policy leaves an excessive number of drug market failures on the table, because there is lack of encouragement

6. Dranove (1998).
7. Scherer and Ross (1990).

of the right kinds of research and development under existing patent law. There are far too many beneficial medications and treatments that could be developed, but are not being developed, and conversely a surfeit of drugs being produced and sold at prices that, in hindsight, may not be socially justified. The fundamental problem is that the current system of drug patent protection and pricing still leaves an underproduction of knowledge regarding the relative benefits and costs of alternative treatments. The focus of drug manufacturers is on marketing products quickly, getting patentable medications through the FDA approval process with short-term, placebo-controlled clinical trials using small patient samples and surrogate laboratory markers as proxies for endpoints. This means that allocation of scarce pharmaceutical research and development and marketing resources is often skewed toward therapies that would not fare nearly as well if relatively small amounts were invested in new knowledge creation beyond the short-term surrogate markers to determine hard clinical endpoints. This also means that resources are taken away from proving the value of therapies that may have enormous social benefit but little profit potential under existing patent law.

Because the current drug pricing and patent system underproduces outcome evidence, price index measurement of drug price inflation is highly problematic. Suppose two new drugs appear on the market and each costs 10 percent more than the weighted average of existing medications in their therapeutic class. One of these medications has unknown fatal side effects that will lead the FDA to pull it off the market in five years. The other medication saves innumerable lives, but this fact is not fully recognized, since only short-term clinical trial evidence is available, and this evidence only establishes the drug's effect on surrogate clinical markers. If both products become widely used, price indexes will need to reflect how much of the increase in drug expenditures reflects pure price increase and how much reflects medical outcome changes. But, as we will argue is the case of many real-world examples, the medical outcomes from drug treatment in this hypothetical example are either unknown or only partially or incorrectly known. Price index theory assumes that consumers actually know which items belong in their market basket of purchases. In the case of pharmaceuticals, this assumption is often not valid.

How should those who calculate price indexes identify the changes in drug expenditures that are due to quality or quantity differences rather than pure price changes? Although it would be preferable to always have objective measures of drug outcomes, price index calculation of drug outcomes are often not well established. A simple approach would be to use whatever people who buy drugs think outcomes are at that time. Thus if many doctors prescribed a hypothetical drug with fatal side effects until it was pulled from the market, this would then mean that their incorrect assessment of the medication's value is nevertheless the measure of outcomes that should be used in computing a price index. This approach implies that those calculating price indexes would have to establish and maintain a database of the clinician-perceived comparative effects of drugs on patient prognosis, quality of life, and recovery from illness, and how these perceptions change over time. This database would presumably have to periodically capture and aggregate the varying opinions of different prescribers in some meaningful way.

This would be a difficult and complex research agenda to implement. Suppose a new oral diabetes drug, drug D, costing 50 percent more than the use-weighted average for existing oral diabetes medications, is approved by the FDA. Suppose further that it immediately captures half of the diabetes oral medication market because it has demonstrated tighter serum glucose control and fewer side effects than older medications, in short-term placebo-controlled clinical trials. How much of the 25 percent increase in diabetes medication expenditure is pure increase in drug D's price, how much is improvement in patient daily quality of life, and how much is expected benefit in lower future health care costs or reduction in diabetic disease complications?

Each prescribing clinician's assessment of the outcomes associated with this new medication and the comparative effects of other oral medications would need to be assessed and averaged to estimate the pure price and "outcome" components of the changed drug price index. Presumably, because of data collection costs, only a representative sample of practicing clinicians would be surveyed for this analysis. How would clinicians' outcome assessment be aggregated? Those clinicians who projected improved outcomes with the new expensive medication would be the most likely to prescribe it, whereas those who did not switch would have a less favorable opinion of its outcomes, benefits, and price. We might take the equivalent dose prescription-weighted average of survey prescriber opinions on medication outcomes (for all prescribers of diabetes medications), but then we would still need clinical agreement on dose equivalency among drugs from possibly very different therapeutic categories. Suppose that those who prescribed drug D thought, on average, that only half the dose of drug D was equivalent to the standard dose of other drugs, while those who prescribed other oral diabetes drugs thought, on average, that a full dose of drug D was needed for equivalency. Suppose that each clinician had different views of standard dose equivalency based on the patient's diabetes severity and use of insulin. The basis for developing an appropriately weighted assessment of medication outcomes based on current clinician opinion, in the absence of objective information, could easily become chimerical.

One alternative would be to develop drug price indexes that reflected the range of uncertainty regarding outcomes for each drug product included in the market basket. Thus if the plausible range of outcomes for drug D was from (1) no improvement in patient health or reduction in cost beyond existing therapies to (2) a 50 percent reduction in health care treatment and indirect costs of diabetes, the price index calculation would include this range for each of the market basket drugs with uncertain outcomes. A panel of clinical experts could be established to develop the range of outcomes for each medication in the market basket. A solution of this type is bound to be disconcerting to policymakers, since imprecise point estimates are usually preferred to accurate confidence intervals for policy purposes. Moreover, this would introduce a high level of subjectivity in price index calculation. Methods for choosing clinical experts to make outcomes decisions could create bias or the appearance of bias in price index calculations.

A third alternative would be to develop objective measures of drug outcomes for each pharmaceutical product. This would also be a difficult research agenda.

Failures of Pharmaceutical Patent Protection

It is not widely understood why so little is known about the actual outcomes associated with many of the most important pharmaceuticals and drug categories. We will present a number of examples that underscore this point. The lack of knowledge has a huge societal cost and broad implications for the evidentiary basis for medical decisionmaking. It certainly complicates drug price index calculation. Subsequently, we will propose a simple extension of current patent law that would deal with many of the shortcomings that we have identified in our examples. The "use-patent" proposal would have the added benefits of providing much better objective data on drug outcomes, enhancing informed consumer choice, and simplifying price index calculation.

Vitamin E and Aspirin

Consider a drug manufacturer trying to decide whether to invest $100 million in a research and development program for a new cardiovascular medication (an A-2 antihypertensive medication, say) or to invest the same resources in research and development for vitamin E (alpha-tocopherol) to prevent heart disease. The new antihypertensive medication is patented and might generate several hundred million dollars in annual revenue if successful, whereas the vitamin E trial would generate essentially no revenue for the manufacturer, since vitamin E is nonpatentable, widely available from numerous manufacturers, and sold over the counter without prescription, as a commodity item.

Current scientific evidence suggests that vitamin E, a potent antioxidant, may have the ability to reduce cardiovascular disease by 25 percent.[8] This would make it one of the most important cardiovascular preventive therapies available, possibly more clinically beneficial than aspirin, antithrombolytic therapy, surgical revascularization, smoking cessation, antihypertensive medications, lipid-lowering medications, diet, or exercise. If vitamin E were as efficacious as some believe, the potential annual U.S. benefits in reduced direct and indirect costs of cardiovascular disease of establishing this fact would exceed $25 billion.[9] Vitamin E has also been suggested to have favorable effects on some types of cancer as well as on Alzheimer's disease.[10]

Scientific speculation regarding vitamin E's potential benefits has existed for nearly three decades. Should vitamin E ultimately be proved to have clinical value in preventing heart disease and in other applications, more than half a trillion dollars in unnecessary health care and economic productivity may have been lost in the United States alone because of the inability of drug companies to capitalize financially by turning promising scientific speculation into pivotal clinical trials.

Aspirin is another example. It has been recognized for nearly fifty years that the antithrombolytic effects of aspirin may benefit heart attack and stroke victims. But there has been little profit in aspirin, a generic over-the-counter product, and no way for a profit-seeking company to justify expansion of the aspirin market by conducting rigorous clinical trials to demonstrate the benefits of aspirin. When the studies to establish

8. Rimm and others (1993); Stampfer and others (1993); and Stephens and others (1996).
9. American Heart Association (1996).
10. Bendich, Mallick, and Leader (1997); Ghadirian and others (1997); and Sano and others (1997).

these clinical benefits were finally conducted by the National Institutes of Health (NIH) in the 1980s, patients had been suffering unnecessary cardiovascular diseases and deaths for more than three decades.[11] Even today, not all heart attack survivors are prescribed aspirin when clinically indicated, because in dramatic comparison to the marketing launch of a patented drug, new information regarding the benefits of aspirin percolates slowly to providers and patients when the pill is a commodity item. The failure of drug pricing policies to reward socially relevant pharmaceutical research and development in these two cases may have cost the United States many times the value of all currently marketed cardiovascular medications and all taxpayer monies spent by the NIH since its inception.

Dranove has looked at the issue of NIH funding of vitamin E studies in some detail.[12] Taking into account current uncertainties about the uncertain payoffs, he finds that the benefit-cost ratio of additional NIH-funded research on vitamin E ranges from 2:1 to 500:1. After concluding that NIH funding in this area is inadequate, he speculates that this is due either to a bias of NIH in favor of curative rather than preventive interventions or to inefficient allocation of research funds within NIH. He rejects the free-rider underprovision of public goods answer, since the societal expected net payoff of additional vitamin E research would be positive for the United States alone even if other countries took advantage of the findings.

Anti-Ulcer Medication

Peptic ulcer disease (PUD) affects more than 5 million Americans at any one time and has been estimated to cost $5.6 billion annually.[13] For the past two decades, histamine2-receptor antagonists (H2RAs) were the treatment of choice for PUD. These medications (cimetidine, ranitidine, famotidine, and nizatidine), until recently available only by prescription, quickly became the highest-selling medications in history, with annual worldwide sales in the billions of dollars.[14] Smith-Kline Beecham's profits from cimetidine sales in the early 1980s accounted for a large portion of total pharmaceutical industry profits in many of those years.[15] Glaxo-

11. Physician's Health Study Research Group, Steering Committee (1989).
12. Dranove (1998).
13. Sonnenberg and Everhart (1997).
14. Pharmaceutical Information Associates (1997).
15. Grabowski and Vernon (1990).

Wellcome's ranitidine went on to become the world pharmaceutical sales and profit leader for more than a decade.

With *Helicobacter pylori* now fully established as a significant etiologic pathogen in PUD, there has been a major shift in the treatment.[16] Although symptomatic therapy is still employed, treatment now includes aggressive eradication of the *H. pylori* bacteria from the gastrointestinal tract using garden-variety generic antibiotics such as metronidazole, tetracycline, and amoxicillin, which cost pennies per treatment. Prior to the recognition of *H. pylori* as a crucial pathogen in the PUD disease process, patients typically suffered periods of ten to fifteen years of active disease and remission.[17]

H. pylori eradication with generic antibiotics was first speculated as being a valid approach to reducing PUD in the early 1980s, just as H2RA sales were beginning to skyrocket.[18] Because generic antibiotic therapy had little profit potential, it took fifteen more years, and tens of billions of dollars spent on unnecessary PUD maintenance therapy, for clinical research to establish the validity of *H. pylori* eradication with antibiotics. By apparent coincidence, the medical community began to start adopting antibiotic treatment for PUD just at the time when H2RAs were losing patent protection and were being relaunched and repositioned as over-the-counter bromides for pepperoni pizza overdose.

Diabetes Therapy

Diabetes mellitus is one of the most expensive diseases in the United States, with direct costs estimated at $91.2 billion and indirect costs of $46.6 billion annually ($137.7 billion total).[19] The American Diabetic Association estimates that 16 million Americans have diabetes. Of these, 8 million patients have been formally diagnosed and know that they have the disease; the other 8 million are undiagnosed. In 1993, approximately 400,000 deaths from all causes are estimated to have occurred in people with diabetes. This represents 5 percent of all persons known to have diabetes and 18 percent of all deaths in the United States in persons aged twenty-five years and older.[20]

16. Soll (1996).
17. Neil (1997).
18. Marshall and Warren (1984).
19. Rubin, Altman, and Mendelson (1994).
20. National Center for Health Statistics (1994)

Given the enormous economic burden of diabetes, it is astonishing how little is known about long-term effectiveness of existing oral diabetes therapy. It is not uncommon practice in American medicine for the FDA to approve medications, and for doctors to prescribe medications, solely on the basis of short-term safety and efficacy studies using surrogate laboratory markers (for example, serum glucose levels) to evaluate clinical benefit. Thus, if oral therapy is demonstrated to maintain a patient's serum glucose within normal range, it is generally assumed that the medication is beneficial to the patient for what really matters, namely, to reduce macro- and microvascular complications of diabetes mellitus such as coronary heart disease, retinopathy, nephropathy, and peripheral neuropathy.

The pivotal diabetes therapy intervention study, the Diabetes Control and Complications Trial (DCCT), evaluated subjects with insulin-dependent diabetes mellitus (IDDM). Also known as juvenile diabetes or hereditary diabetes, IDDM affects about 5 percent of the diabetic population. DCCT demonstrated that tight control of glucose levels with insulin injections reduces diabetes-related long-term complications.[21] On the other hand, non-insulin-dependent diabetes mellitus (NIDDM) represents 95 percent of the population and is a major economic burden to society. Although it seems logical to apply the long-term benefits of tight metabolic control using insulin in IDDM to NIDDM, the University Group Diabetes Program (UGDP) study of NIDDM showed no clinical benefit of insulin and sulfonylurea therapy.[22] The study also suggested tolbutamide, a first generation sulfonylurea, may actually increase the incidence of cardiovascular deaths. Since the sample size of this study may be too small to make any definitive conclusion, the United Kingdom Prospective Diabetes Study (UKPDS) was initiated in 1977 to examine the effect of diet, insulin, oral hypoglycemic agents such as metformin and glyburide on long-term outcomes of diabetic patients. Preliminary results of this study, such as the effect of treatment on metabolic control, have been published; however, the results have been disappointing, with marginal improvement in the average HgbA1c when hypoglycemic agents are compared to dietary therapy. Diabetes control actually deteriorates over the nine-year follow-up period, suggesting disease progression despite hypoglycemic therapy. Macrovascular disease such as coro-

21. Diabetes Control and Complications Trial Research Group (1993).
22. "Effects of Hypoglycemic Agents on Vascular Complications in Patients with Adult-Onset Diabetes" (1982).

nary artery disease also occurred in 20 percent of the study patients, with fatal outcomes due to macrovascular disease occurring seventy times more frequently than among patients with microvascular disease.[23] Given the small improvement in glycemic control observed with treatment, it is uncertain whether substantial long-term benefits, especially prevention of macrovascular disease, will be revealed in the UKPDS study. The study just ended in 1998. It is important to recognize that despite the availability and use of hypoglycemic agents to treat NIDDM for numerous decades, no long-term studies in NIDDM patients have been able to show the benefit of these agents in preventing or delaying diabetic complications.[24] The results of the UKPDS study will have significant impact on how we allocate our health care resources. As the UKPDS investigators have suggested, if therapy to improve glucose control is shown to be ineffective in maintaining health, one should reserve the huge amount of health care resources that we currently spend on medications and intensive glucose monitoring for other more cost-effective therapies, for example, screening for diabetic complications and other cardiovascular risk factors such as hypertension, dyslipidemia, and smoking.

One might argue that outcome studies like the UKPDS should have been conducted long before the approval of oral hypoglycemic agents for the management of NIDDM. Drug companies are extremely reluctant to pursue such outcome research for two reasons. First, the studies are not needed to market the medications. Second, the studies could cost tens of millions of dollars, take many years to complete, and might actually demonstrate limited benefits, side effects, or even harm for some of the medications. No pharmaceutical executive motivated by quarterly corporate earnings reports is going to endear himself or herself to Wall Street analysts by proposing a ten-year study to establish whether the company's diabetes medication actually works (long after the drug's patent has expired).

Antihypertensive Therapy

Hypertension (high blood pressure) is common throughout the world and is a major public health and medical problem. Hypertension is usually asymptomatic; however, symptoms such as headache on wakening, blurred vision, and dizziness can occur in patients who have very high blood pressure (for example, hypertensive urgency or emergency). Hy-

23. United Kingdom Prospective Diabetes Study Group (1996).
24. Wolffenbuttel and Haeften (1995).

pertension is also a major risk factor for coronary artery disease, stroke, and cardiovascular death. About 50 million Americans are known to have elevated blood pressure (systolic blood pressure of 140 mm Hg or greater or diastolic blood pressure of 90 mm Hg or higher) or are taking antihypertensive medications.[25] The annual U.S. costs of treating hypertension-related cardiovascular events can be estimated at approximately $60 billion.[26]

More Americans meet current indications for antihypertensive medication than any other life-threatening condition, and this therapeutic class is the most frequently prescribed.[27] Nonetheless, the evidence showing the actual benefits to patients for the vast majority of antihypertensive medicines is weak or nonexistent. It has been rigorously shown that low-dose thiazide diuretics (specifically, hydrochlorthiazide plus amiloride, chlorthalidone) and beta blockers (atenolol, metoprolol, pindolol) reduce cardiovascular morbidity and mortality in isolated systolic hypertension and hypertension in the elderly.[28] No long-term outcome studies have been done with other antihypertensives, including the loop diuretics, calcium channel blockers, ACE inhibitors, or alpha blockers, to show their effects on cardiovascular disease mortality. It is well known that different antihypertensives have differing levels of efficacy in patients with different demographics and comorbid conditions (for example, diabetes, hyperlipidemia, kidney failure, existing heart disease).[29] It has also been established that there are significant quality-of-life differences between antihypertensive medications within the same ACE-inhibitor therapeutic class (for example, enalapril and captopril).[30] Nevertheless, with the exception of a few beta blockers and low-dose thiazide diuretics, all of the evidence supporting drug use is based on short-term clinical trials using control of blood pressure as a surrogate marker for disease benefits rather than data on the effectiveness of these medications in reducing patient morbidity and mortality.

There is some evidence that antihypertensive medications are not uniformly beneficial to patients and that some patients may have been harmed by some of these drugs. For instance, the use of non-potassium-

25. "The Fifth Report of the Joint National Committee on the Detection, Evaluation, and Treatment of High Blood Pressure" (1993).

26. Grimm (1989).

27. National Center for Health Statistics (1996).

28. Curb and others (1996); Dahlot and others (1991); and Medical Research Council (1992).

29. Carter and others (1994).

30. Testa and others (1993).

sparing diuretics such as loop diuretics and high-dose thiazide diuretics has been associated with increased risk of sudden cardiac death in a selected group of hypertensive individuals.[31] Recent epidemiological studies have also demonstrated 60 percent increased risk for myocardial infarction associated with the use of short-acting calcium channel blockers such as nifedipine.[32] Recent publication of the results of the Appropriate Blood Pressure Control in Diabetes (ABCD) trial further suggested the need for long-term outcome evidence of calcium channel blockers in the management of hypertension. The ABCD trial is a five-year randomized, blinded study comparing the efficacy of nisoldipine with enalapril in the management of hypertension in patients with diabetes mellitus.[33] The use of nisoldipine was found to be associated with higher incidence of nonfatal and fatal myocardial infarctions despite similar blood pressure control as compared with the enalapril treatment group. Several large-scale clinical trials are being conducted to confirm these adverse findings.[34]

In the last decade, none of the pharmaceutical manufacturers has been willing to fund studies to see how effective these various agents are in head-to-head randomized clinical trials powered to detect differences in cardiovascular and mortality endpoints. Long-term outcome studies were not initiated until adverse outcomes were demonstrated in epidemiological studies. This huge class of medicines is prescribed to millions of Americans essentially on faith.

Anti-Arrhythmia Therapy

Arrhythmias are irregular heartbeats or rhythms due to abnormal impulse conduction or formation in cardiac cells. Although the presence of arrhythmia is a well-described risk factor for sudden cardiac death, suppression of these abnormal impulses using anti-arrhythmic agents has not been shown to be beneficial. In 1991, the National Institutes of Health launched the Cardiac Arrhythmia Suppression Trial (CAST) to assess the benefits of flecainide, encainide, and moricizine, a class of anti-arrhythmic medications, in the management of arrhythmias in post-myocardial infarction survivors.[35] Ten months after initiation of the

---

31. Grobbee and Hoes (1995).
32. Furberg and Psaty (1995).
33. Estacio and others (1998).
34. ALLHAT Research Group 1996); and NORDIL Group (1993).
35. Cardiac Arrhythmia Suppression Trial Investigators (1989); Cardiac Arrhythmia Suppression Trial II Investigators (1992).

study, the CAST was discontinued due to excess cardiac arrests and total mortality in treated patients. The CAST study raised many concerns about chronic use of anti-arrhythmic agents. Although it is logical to assume that short-term use of antiarrhythmic agents to abort arrhythmias may improve symptoms and cardiac function, long-term use of these agents to suppress irregular rhythm formation is not without harm. Antiarrhythmic agents such as quinidine and procainamide are pro-arrhythmic, which means that these agents can induce more arrhythmias. Other agents such as disopyramide can make ventricular function worse and can precipitate congestive heart failure in patients with underlying heart disease. So far, none of the FDA-approved antiarrhythmic agents have been shown to reduce cardiac mortality. Therefore, longer-term studies to investigate the real benefit of this group of agents are necessary.

Lipid Therapy

When it comes to rigorously demonstrating the value of drug therapy in reducing mortality and morbidity, cholesterol lowering medications, particularly the statins (HMG Co-A reductase inhibitors), represent a uniquely positive situation in pharmaceutical outcomes research. More clinical trial information has been collected for the statins than for any other therapy in history. At this point, more than 200,000 patient-years of randomized placebo-controlled clinical trial data on statin therapy exist. We now know that pravastatin is effective in reducing cardiovascular disease and mortality in primary prevention for hypercholesterolemic patients (WOSCOPS study), and in reducing mortality and preventing secondary disease in cardiovascular disease patients with or without hypercholesterolemia (LIPID and CARE studies).[36] We also know that simvastatin is effective in reducing cardiovascular disease and mortality in hypercholesterolemic patients with pre-existing heart disease (4S study) and that lovastatin is effective in reducing cardiovascular disease in primary prevention for patients without substantially elevated serum cholesterol (AFCAPS/TEXCAPS study).[37] Since all these studies have included dietary recommendations and cardiovascular risk factor counseling in both the treatment and placebo groups, the disease risk reduc-

36. Sacks and others (1996); Shepherd and others (1995); and Tonkin, for the LIPID Study Group (1997).
37. Gotto (1997); and Scandinavian Simvastatin Survival Study group (1994).

tion from statins is additive to the benefits of other cardiovascular therapies and risk factor reduction.

The fact that all these outcomes studies have taken place within this therapeutic category but have not occurred within other disease categories is initially puzzling but probably reflects historical accident. Two earlier studies of cholesterol therapy conducted in the early 1980s, the LRC-CPPT trial of cholestyramine and the Helsinki Heart Study of gemfibrozil, demonstrated that although each of these agents reduced cardiovascular disease, in both studies there was a statistically nonsignificant increase in all-cause mortality among treated patients.[38] Despite assurances to the medical community from many clinical experts that these studies were not powered to detect mortality differences and that these excess-mortality results were merely statistical flukes, some practicing clinicians and academic experts believed that cholesterol reduction therapy may be harmful to patients.

By the late 1980s, Merck, until recently the largest manufacturer of statin therapy (simvastatin-Zocor, lovastatin-Mevacor), decided to risk a study of the effects of simvastatin on all-cause mortality. This was done to overcome the substantial market resistance to statin therapy, despite its apparently high level of short-term safety, patient acceptability, and tolerability. They chose to conduct a double-blind placebo-controlled study in an extremely high-risk hypercholesterolemic study population from Scandinavia with pre-existing coronary artery disease. Scandinavia was chosen because its incidence of heart disease and cardiovascular death was among the highest in the world, facilitating a study designed specifically for detection of mortality differences. The study results were highly favorable, showing a relative risk reduction in all-cause mortality of 30 percent in the simvastatin treatment ($p = 0.0003$).

In response to the initiation of the 4S study, and based on some surprisingly favorable small-sample clinical trial results for their statin product (pravastatin-Pravachol), Bristol-Myers Squibb initiated a series of large-scale cardiovascular outcomes studies to document the benefits of pravastatin. Although the 4S study results were not yet in, Bristol-Myers Squibb had little to lose by taking these clinical trial research risks. In fact, they had no choice. Had they refused to do outcomes research and the 4S results turned out favorably for Merck's simvastatin, they would have been left out in the cold with a drug that was not as potent in

---

38. Frick and others (1987); Lipid Research Clinics Program (1984a, 1984b).

lowering cholesterol as simvastatin and without outcomes evidence supporting pravastatin for reduction of mortality and cardiovascular disease. If the simvastatin 4S results turned out badly, lack of outcome data for pravastatin would mean that they would be tarred with the same brush. As it happened, all of the pravastatin studies showed highly favorable results in reducing cardiovascular disease and mortality. The pravastatin WOSCOPS results showed a reduction in clinical events that was approximately 50 percent higher than would have been predicted from Framingham epidemiological projections on the benefits of reducing cholesterol values in the U.S. population.[39] As a result of these trials, it is now widely thought in the cardiology community that pravastatin, and possibly other statins, may have clinical benefits in cardiovascular disease reduction that are not fully characterized by the therapy's effectiveness in altering surrogate lipid markers (HDL, LDL, total serum cholesterol, triglycerides).[40] Until these studies were completed, it was an article of faith in the medical community that altering the profile of lipids circulating in the bloodstream was the only mechanism that mattered for cholesterol therapy to prevent heart disease.

The history of the statin market shows that pharmaceutical companies can easily carry out rigorous outcome research for their products when motivated to do so. Why did they do it for statins but not for antihypertensives, H2RAs, diabetes medications, or vitamin E? We think that the world owes a vast research debt to the six extra people who died in the LRC study treatment group and the seven extra people who died in the Helsinki Heart Study treatment group.[41] Had these random fatal events not occurred, we doubt that Merck would have faced the same resistance to statin market growth that led them to sponsor the 4S study. Without the 4S study, Bristol-Myers Squibb would not have seen an obligation to respond by demonstrating rigorously that pravastatin, although not as potent in lowering serum cholesterol as simvastatin, was at least as effective in preventing cardiovascular disease and death.

Unfortunately, now that these studies have been released and the medical community is reassured that the statin safety and efficacy profiles are legitimate, many clinicians have gone right back to the assumption that surrogate lipid markers are all that matters. A new statin, released in 1997 by Parke-Davis and Pfizer (atorvastatin), has had one of the most

39. WOSCOPS Study Group (in press).
40. Shepherd (1997).
41. Wysowski and Gross (1990).

successful pharmaceutical product launches in history with annual sales reaching $1 billion in less than one year. There are no outcome study data available for atorvastatin at all—only surrogate marker data. But it is the most potent cholesterol agent in the category, and it produces pretty patient medical charts.[42]

Taxol

Taxol (the branded version of paclitaxel) was developed by the National Cancer Institute in the 1980s. Since the federal government does not market drugs, a standard NIH marketing arrangement—a Collaborative Research and Development Agreement (CRADA)—was competitively bid for by the drug industry. Bristol-Myers Squibb acquired a five-year marketing exclusivity agreement for Taxol expiring in December 1997. The introduction of paclitaxel was an important milestone in cancer chemotherapy, since it offers better survival and cost-effective treatment for some cancers. Currently, Taxol is approved for refractory breast and ovarian cancer and Kaposi's sarcoma.[43] Clinical research has demonstrated the utility of Taxol in enhancing patient survival for these indications. Clinical trials are under way to support Taxol use for a number of other indications, such as head and neck and first-line breast cancer.[44]

A recent consultant report said that extending current Taxol marketing exclusivity for two years would cost Americans $1.3 billion.[45] Based on extrapolating trends from other chemotherapy drugs that have already lost patent protection (Megace, VePesid, Hydrea, Mutamycin), however, their figures show that 73 percent of this increased expenditure would be due to expanded Taxol use (not higher Taxol prices) by patients meeting current and future indications for the drug. Prior experience with these other chemotherapeutic agents suggests that after a cancer drug goes generic, research for new uses ceases, companies stop actively promoting current uses, and doctors are no longer actively detailed by pharmaceutical sales representatives. For these reasons, historical evidence suggests that use of the branded chemotherapeutic agents can actually be higher than it would be with generic competition.

Should marketing exclusivity for Taxol be eliminated after five years? After all, this was a medicine developed by the government at taxpayer

42. Bakker-Arkema and others (1996).
43. Hortobagyi and others (1997); McGuire and others (1996); and Saville and others (1995).
44. Fountzilas and others (1997); and Meerpohl and others (1997).
45. Max (1997).

expense. Why should a big pharmaceutical company obtain additional monopoly price protection for it?

The answer may not be as simple as it seems. There are no obviously superior therapies available for the tumor types that meet current or expected Taxol indications. Even under generic competition, paclitaxel will be a relatively expensive chemotherapeutic regimen because of its specific manufacturing requirements. If, as has happened with other chemotherapeutic agents, patients who would have benefited from Taxol are switched to cheaper drugs that are not as effective, the costs to society could be large. Following historic trends, it can be projected that nearly 200,000 patient-years of life would be lost in the next seven years as patients are switched from generic paclitaxel to other less effective chemotherapies, and as clinical trials for new indications are less vigorously pursued by generic manufacturers.[46] Assuming that each of these years of life are worth at least $20,000 to the patients and their families, the net loss to society could exceed $2.8 billion, even after accounting for the increased price of Taxol treatment with two years of extended marketing exclusivity.

Periodontal Disease

Periodontal disease, a common source of tooth loss, results from dental plaque, a combination of bacteria and sticky bacterial products that forms on the teeth. When left to accumulate, the proportion of harmful bacterial species in dental plaque grows and begins to damage surrounding tissues. Plaque resulting in inflammation or infection of the gums is called gingivitis; that of the bone, periodontitis. Periodontitis is treated either by surgically eliminating periodontal pockets or by cleaning affected tooth roots in a process known as scaling and planing.[47]

It has been suggested for several decades that systemic or topical chemotherapeutic prophylaxis to control harmful bacteria would be superior to surgical or mechanical intervention alone.[48] Research progress has been extremely slow, in large part because the antibiotics (for example, metronidazole) used to control periodontal plaque are generic, cheap, and not likely to generate any significant profit for those demonstrating this use.

46. Hay and others (1998).
47. FDA Consumer Website (1990).
48. Formicola, Gottsegan, and Hay (1981).

In recent NIH-funded studies, Loesche and others compared scaling and root planing plus placebo medication (positive control) with scaling and root planing plus metronidazole (test) for their ability to treat advanced forms of periodontal disease. Among patients seen at an inner city hospital they found that 90 percent of the periodontal surgical needs could be avoided with the metronidazole treatment.[49] Loesche indicates that these studies "seem to have been either ignored or dismissed by the clinical and academic community." Ironically, if metronidazole were a patented antibiotic, the manufacturer would almost certainly put substantial marketing resources into convincing the clinical community that antibiotic treatment of periodontal disease was less invasive, cost-effective, cosmetically superior, and less risky than surgery.

Use Patents: A Modest Proposal for Market Reform

Fen-Phen, anyone?[50] All of these examples suggest serious market failure, and they are not atypical. Let us be clear that we are not criticizing pharmaceutical companies for maximizing profits under the current legal and regulatory constraints but rather the constraints themselves. Pharmaceutical research with very high potential social benefit and modest cost is usually not pursued when the returns cannot be privately appropriated. This pattern cannot be expected to change as long as current patent law provides the main property rights protection for pharmaceutical research and development. If anything, the NIH and other public agencies bear most of the blame for the current state of affairs. They are responsible for developing valuable public information when the market is incapable of doing so. The fact that so many important clinical issues are being researched so slowly by the public sector suggests that government spending may not be the solution either.

The key problem is that patents protect products, not medical treatments. They do not encourage appropriate use of these products prior to patent expiration and provide no incentive to generate new knowledge once the drug patent expires. The FDA grants marketing approval for new medications based on short-term safety and efficacy studies. These studies often use surrogate clinical markers of disease endpoints because it is much easier and cheaper to show that a drug reduces blood pressure,

49. Loesche and others (1996).
50. Patalas and others (1997); Connolly and others (1997).

cholesterol, or serum glucose, for example, than to demonstrate that the drug actually reduces heart disease, stroke, kidney disease, or mortality. With average drug development times already exceeding a decade, the financial pressures to bring a product to market based on short-term studies are enormous. Pharmaceutical manufacturers concentrate on short-term studies that are most likely to get the drug approved by the FDA as quickly as possible rather than on costlier studies that follow many more patients over much longer periods of time to document the true outcome effects on patient morbidity and mortality.

Once a drug is on the market and is generating adequate revenue, there is little incentive to do the additional research necessary to show whether it actually works rather than just generates a pretty surrogate lab test profile. It is true that the FDA will expand a drug's marketing indications after successful demonstration of disease reduction benefits, but this incentive is woefully inadequate. A risk-averse pharmaceutical executive does not think twice about taking a decision to halt or severely limit research at the drug marketing approval point, regardless of the potential social benefits of demonstrating actual patient outcomes. If the drug were to ultimately show disease reduction benefits, these would come at high cost and often after several years of effort (often after patent expiration), reducing the drug's postmarketing profitability, and would then merely confirm what everyone thought to begin with.

If outcome studies were known to be under way, some in the medical community would use the excuse of waiting until the evidence was actually in before prescribing the medication. If there were no outcome studies under way, clinicians would have to bite the bullet, and many would decide to use the product. In the absence of studies proving disease benefits, pharmaceutical companies can find ways to market the implied hard clinical endpoint benefits of therapy without actually guaranteeing that these benefits occur.

What if the outcome studies showed that the drug was not very effective in reducing disease, or was actually harmful? It is difficult and expensive enough to get any product through FDA approval and successful market launch. An unfavorable postmarketing outcome study could halt or reduce product revenues and, if bad enough, even generate multimillion-dollar lawsuits. If such an outcomes study had never occurred, the medication would have been a net contributor to corporate profits. After the bad news was in, any drug company executive that had authorized such an outcomes study would be quickly asked to exercise their corpo-

rate parachute option (golden or lead), having turned a perfectly successful product into a financial nightmare.

The Use-Patent Proposal

If, instead, patent law were enhanced to provide some period of marketing exclusivity protection for specific proven uses of medications,
rather than just the product itself, the level and allocation of pharmaceutical research and development would improve dramatically. Anyone
could apply for this "use-patent" protection, regardless of whether the
drug was protected by a standard product patent or not. If the applicant
were the first to demonstrate to regulators (for example, the FDA) that
the drug had specific clinical benefits, it would be granted marketing
exclusivity for that specific use of the product for some period of time,
say, five years, even if it did not hold the original product patent on that
medication.

The regulators would decide how broad the use patents would be,
given the quality and comprehensiveness of the supporting evidence. The
use patents would be hierarchical. For example, an applicant that demonstrated proven benefits of a lipid product in reducing heart disease
would be granted marketing exclusivity over an applicant that had merely
shown that the drug lowered serum cholesterol. This is because it can
reasonably be presumed that the only motive for lowering serum cholesterol is to reduce the risk of cardiovascular disease. A third applicant who
demonstrated the benefits of this therapy in reducing all-cause mortality
would preempt the heart disease reduction use patent, since it can be
reasonably presumed that the primary motivation for reducing risk of
heart disease is to reduce mortality risk.

The use patents would be complementary. For example, an applicant
that demonstrated the benefits of the lipid therapy in reducing stroke
would receive use-patent protection for patients prescribed the medication to prevent stroke rather than heart disease, even if a heart disease
use patent were already in force for the medication. On the other hand,
since the primary motive for avoiding stroke is also to reduce mortality
risk, an all-cause mortality risk reduction use patent would preempt the
stroke use patent as well as the heart disease use patent. Some use-patent
protection decisions would inevitably involve regulatory judgment. For
example, if one applicant demonstrated mortality reduction for a drug,
while another demonstrated improvement in daily patient function or
quality of life, it would be up to the regulators to decide whether one use

was superior or complementary to the other use. In some cases, it might be appropriate for applicants to share or cross-license use patents where there was some potential for overlap, but these issues could generally be worked out in the marketplace rather than by the regulatory authority.

The use patents could be expanded or narrowed based on new categorical evidence. Suppose, for example, the first applicant for a lipid product use patent only demonstrated its benefits for reducing heart disease in white men. A second applicant who showed that the drug also reduced heart disease in women, children, or nonwhite ethnic groups could successfully have the original use patent narrowed and obtain use patent protection for marketing to people in those additional demographic categories.

Physicians and other drug prescribers would be required by law to state on their prescription orders the specific intended use of the medication, regardless of whether the drugs were single-source (under standard patent protection), generic, or over-the-counter. Although likely to generate enormous provider resistance even from a clinical perspective, it seems reasonable to document why the drug was being prescribed. Prescriber misrepresentation of treatment purpose would be subject to the same financial and other sanctions that any patent violation would engender. This step of requiring explicit justification for drug orders would, in itself, be a major enhancement in encouraging evidence-based medical practice.

Application of Use Patents

Use patents would not replace existing patents. If an applicant successfully obtained a use patent on a drug under standard patent protection, the applicant would still have to obtain the product from the original patent-holder at whatever price the original patent-holder demanded. There would be obvious research and marketing economies of scale and strategic incentives for the original product patent-holder to carry out vigorous use-patent research to protect its profits, since it would have the largest original knowledge base regarding the product's development and potential ultimate benefits. But it would no longer have the luxury of sitting back and forcing health care decisionmakers to gamble that the drug actually worked in patients, since doing so would allow someone else who actually demonstrated these benefits to grab a large portion of the potential profits.

Use patents could be obtained on generic and over-the-counter products as well as patented products. In this case, the successful use-patent applicant would be granted temporary marketing exclusivity for a specific use of a drug, even when the product had been on the market for many years. Anyone purchasing the product for the specific protected use would have to pay the use-patent-holder for the product rather than obtain the drug at its generic price. To encourage new research rather than opportunistic land grabs for existing knowledge, there would be a grandfather clause exempting all current FDA-approved indications for all marketed products, generic or patented, from use-patent protection. There would still be a major profit incentive for companies to continue research to prove benefits beyond existing indications and to pursue new indications for drugs such as Taxol, even at the point where they are losing marketing exclusivity.

Under use-patent protection, the market would sort out actual drug value much more efficiently than at present. The moment scientific information began to suggest that a specific clinical indication could potentially generate successful patient outcomes, there would be a competitive rush to obtain the use patent. Suppose, however, that experts expected an approved product in a specific therapeutic category to be inferior to competitors. In this case little research to establish its use patents would be carried out, and it would end up with a much smaller set of proven indications than medications that were felt to have superior clinical value. The evidentiary bar within any specific therapeutic category would be continually ratcheted higher as each new use patent was established. To establish subsequent use patents with other medications, it would no longer be ethical to perform placebo-controlled trials, or narrow clinical indication trials, but rather only trials against existing proven therapies in their most comprehensive proven uses. This would continuously tighten the level of evidence needed for every drug to establish and maintain successful market share and make the production of drug outcomes evidence an ongoing dynamic process rather than stagnate at the FDA approval point.

Use Patents: Potential Criticisms

A reasonable criticism of this proposal is that enforcement of use patents would be more complicated and difficult than enforcement of product patents. This is true, but enforcement costs have to be weighed against the potential societal benefits of expanded pharmaceutical knowledge. The enforcement issue is not quite as difficult as some might think. If, for example, a firm successfully obtained a use patent for vitamin E in the prevention of heart attack, it would be clearly impossible to prevent every possible patient from buying standard over-the-counter vitamin E for that use, even without a doctor's prescription. However, if there were a doctor's prescription for vitamin E, there would be a clear trail of evidence that the patient should be receiving the brand of vitamin E protected by use patent. If there were no doctor's prescription for vitamin E (because, for example, the doctor was encouraging the patient to save money by purchasing brands not protected by use patent), the doctor could be sued for failure to provide community standard of care. Doctors would be very reluctant to participate in schemes to avoid use-patent protection because their malpractice premiums would skyrocket.

Just as we recognize that computer software copyright is not perfect protection, we do not abandon it because it occasionally fails. To do so would guarantee a huge reduction in software research and development. Although it would be impossible to prevent every infringement of pharmaceutical use patents, the situation would be analogous to copyright protection of videotapes and disks and probably much more controllable than software piracy. Suppose a large health plan failed to monitor and enforce use patents by its health care providers and patients. As the deep pocket, they would be vulnerable to lawsuits, just as a large corporation that encourages or ignores employee software piracy would be sued now, even though an individual employee or consumer can occasionally sneak copies without being caught.

Some will argue that government, perhaps through expanded funding to the NIH, is the only appropriate mechanism for research into establishing proven uses for new and existing therapy. We and others argue that the real-world examples described above convincingly counter this view.[51] As with any discretionary item in the federal budget, double-digit expansion of NIH spending is not on the horizon at least until the baby boomer generation is well past retirement age. No matter how large their budget, though, the NIH and other federal agencies may not be able to operate as quickly and responsively in demonstrating pharmaceutical outcomes as would a competitive pharmaceutical industry operating under the profit motive.

Where has the NIH been over the past several decades when conclusively and comprehensively establishing the value to patients of aspirin, vitamin E, specific lipid medications, antihypertensives, anti-arrythmics, oral diabetic medications, ulcer therapies, cancer treatments, and so forth, has been scientifically feasible and certainly justifiable from a social cost-benefit perspective? Past NIH drug outcomes studies, while often extremely scientifically valuable, have poorly tracked social priorities and

51. Dranove (1998); and Ward and Dranove (1995).

have sometimes occurred decades after the original hypothesis of therapeutic benefit or harm. The NIH is limited by competing demands for
medical research initiatives, the micro- and macro-politics of bioscientific
research and development resource allocation decisions across diseases
and therapies, the dogma of prevailing scientific paradigms, the prejudices and political correctness of academic experts, and the red tape of
government bureaucracy.

Implementation of use patents would be trickier than for product
patents. It is fairly straightforward to document originality in the development of a new chemical entity. If six different firms were racing to
prove that a given antihypertensive medication reduced stroke, the use
patent would be awarded to the first to prove this case convincingly to the
regulators. Just as for existing safety and efficacy studies in support of a
new drug application to the FDA, specific requirements would be made
explicit, such as requiring that the applicant support all claims with two
carefully controlled clinical trials. Because the FDA would now potentially be evaluating competing clinical trials for the same medication,
there could be times when data from the first firm to file a claim might be
ruled unacceptable, and a later, more qualified applicant would be
awarded the use patent. A corollary benefit of the use-patent system
would be to encourage the development of a research infrastructure to
undertake real-world clinical outcome studies. This would probably involve strategic partnerships between pharmaceutical manufacturers and
managed health care organizations.

It is not the goal of this proposal to burden the FDA or other regulators with adjudicating detailed hierarchies between competing use patents for minor quality-of-life improvements (for example, the drug improves patient's conversation skills versus improves their golf game). We
would even support limitations of the use-patent proposal to lifesaving
therapies, or to those, plus a small number of obviously major health
status enhancements (recovery of eyesight, use of limbs, mental consciousness, and so forth) if these were needed to garner adequate support
from those concerned with excessive regulatory and enforcement costs.

Discussion and Conclusions

Protection of intellectual property has long been recognized as crucial
to economic growth. The Founding Fathers established patent protection
in Article 1, section 8, of the U.S. Constitution. Product patent protection
laws have allowed innovative drugs with innumerable benefits to man-

kind to become available to the public. But there is room for improvement. There is a good deal of intellectual property in medicine that is not protected under the current system and thus fails to materialize.

The implementation of pharmaceutical use patents would align pharmaceutical research and development expenditures much more closely with what society, health care providers, and individual patients demand. Rather than establishing a minimum level of information to obtain FDA marketing approval, manufacturers would have market-based incentives to prove the benefits of therapy in lives saved and illnesses avoided. Use patents would promote dynamic, responsive creation of drug outcomes studies along those avenues of scientific research thought most likely to generate large expected profits. These would generally be the drug use indications that individuals and markets want most to see documented and proven.

Should such a use-patent system prove effective for encouraging outcomes-based pharmaceutical research and development, there is no reason why similar intellectual property protection could not also be applied to other medical interventions, including surgical and diagnostic techniques, medical treatment practice guidelines, clinical pathways, and disease prevention programs. The medical knowledge production free-rider problem is not unique to pharmaceuticals. It exists in all areas of medical care research and practice. In the current competitive environment for managed health care, there are extremely limited incentives to evaluate or improve patient health care through rigorous outcomes research studies, since competitors can take advantage of any new findings (such as new treatment practice guidelines) without investing in the research. Protecting such intellectual property would open the floodgates of valuable competitive medical research and development.

Finally, the outcomes research that will be fostered by use patents will also have substantial potential benefits in improving clinical understanding of disease and therapeutic interventions. Again, the lipid therapy example is a useful case in point, since more long-term clinical trial data have been generated on these medications than for any other therapeutic category.

When the first atherosclerosis reduction clinical trials with lipid agents were initiated in the mid-1980s, clinicians assumed that the primary pathological mechanism for fatal and nonfatal heart attacks were large atherosclerotic plaques that constricted coronary arteries and blood flow and eventually closed off completely through thrombosis. We might call this the "plumbing paradigm" of heart disease. Snake out the arteries and everything would be good as new. The focus of cardiology research was on surgical revascularization techniques, such as angioplasty and coronary bypass, and medical therapies that would widen these coronary restrictions and make the thrombosis harder to establish.[52] We are now in a post-plumbing paradigm.

The lipid therapy trials indicated that very modest changes in progression or regression of atherosclerotic plaques (narrowing of coronary arteries) were often associated with major changes in incidence of heart attack and heart disease.[53] Resulting directly from these clinical trials, the new post-plumbing paradigm in clinical cardiology is that atherosclerotic plaque stability (resistance to plaque rupture) is the key to prevention of ischemic heart disease. Therapies that enhance stability of the diseased heart vessel wall may be much more important than treatments that merely widen vessel constriction. An entirely new direction of cardiovascular research has been opened up with this enhanced understanding of the mechanisms of heart disease pathology from the lipid therapy outcome studies.

As Arrow pointed out thirty-six years ago, health care is different from other goods and services, in large part because of the uncertain risks of disease and the benefits of treatment.[54] When we look at price variation and price change in TV sets, soybeans, or software, there is a legitimate presumption that although information is not perfect, consumers know approximately what they are buying and that price differences reasonably reflect underlying conditions of consumer preference and producer efficiency. In the pharmaceutical marketplace, the underproduction of knowledge is so vast that not even the best clinicians know what they are bargaining for when they prescribe lifetime medication for chronic diseases.

It is becoming increasingly clear that health expenditure statistics should focus on the total cost of treatments for specific conditions rather than simply the prices for drugs, physician services, or other factor inputs.[55] Policy evaluation of health care expenditures in general, and drug expenditures in particular, requires understanding of how prices, outcomes, and quality of care interact to impact health care spending and patient outcomes.[56] Drug price index statistics depend on accurate de-

---

52. Reder (1997).
53. Pitt and others (1995); and Kinlay and Ganz (1997).
54. Arrow (1963).
55. See Triplett, chapter 7 in this volume.
56. See Frank, Berndt, and Busch, chapter 3 in this volume.

composition of pharmaceutical expenditures into output, quality, and price components.

Unfortunately, the vacuum of clinical knowledge regarding therapeutic outcomes severely limits the accuracy of drug price index statistics. If we want drug prices to meaningfully reflect their impacts on patient lives, we need to know what these impacts are so that the marketplace can value pharmaceutical outcomes appropriately. For relatively modest research and development investments compared to the current costs of bringing drugs to market and for trivial investments relative to the social burden of disease, drug prices could much more accurately reflect their social value. Use patents would go a long way toward addressing the market failures that prevent these investments from occurring.

References

ALLHAT Research Group. 1996. "Rationale and Design for the Antihypertensive and Lipid Lowering Treatment to Prevent Heart Attack Trial (ALLHAT)." *American Journal of Hypertension* 9(4, part 1): 342–60.

American Heart Association. 1996. *Heart and Stroke Facts: 1996 Statistics Supplement.* Dallas: American Heart Association.

Arrow, Kenneth. 1963. "Uncertainty and the Welfare Economics of Medical Care." *American Economic Review* 53 (December): 941–73.

Bakker-Arkema, Rebecca G., and others. 1996. "Efficacy and Safety of a New HMG-CoA Reductase Inhibitor, Atorvastatin, in Patients with Hypertriglyceridemia." *Journal of the American Medical Association* 275(2): 128–33.

Bendich, A., R. Mallick, and S. Leader. 1997. "Potential Health Economic Benefits of Vitamin Supplementation." *Western Journal of Medicine* 166(5): 306–12.

Cardiac Arrhythmia Suppression Trial investigators. 1989. "Preliminary Report: Effect of Encainide and Flecainide on Mortality in a Randomized Trial of Arrhythmia Suppression after Myocardial Infarction." *New England Journal of Medicine* 321(6): 406–12.

Cardiac Arrhythmia Suppression Trial II investigators. 1992. "Effect of the Antiarrhythmic Agent Moricizine on Survival after Myocardial Infarction." *New England Journal of Medicine* 327(4): 227–33.

Carter, Barry L., and others. 1994. "Selected Factors That Influence Responses to Antihypertensives." *Archives of Family Medicine* 3(6): 528–36.

Connolly, H. M., and others. 1997. "Valvular Heart Disease Associated with Fenfluramine-Phentermine." *New England Journal of Medicine* 337(9): 581–88.

Curb, J. D., and others. 1996. "Effect of Diuretic-Based Antihypertensive Treatment on Cardiovascular Disease Risk in Older Diabetic Patients with Isolated Systolic Hypertension: Systolic Hypertension in the Elderly Program Cooperative Research Group." *Journal of the American Medical Association* 276(23): 1886–92.

Dahlof, B., and others. 1991. "Morbidity and Mortality in the Swedish Trial in Old Patients with Hypertension (STOP-HTN)." *Lancet* 338(8778): 1281–85.

Diabetes Control and Complications Trial Research Group. 1993. "The Effect of Intensive Treatment of Diabetes on the Development and Progression of Long-Term Complications in Insulin-Dependent Diabetes Mellitus." *New England Journal of Medicine* 329(14): 977–86.

DiMasi, J. A., and others. 1995. "Research and Development Costs for New Drugs by Therapeutic Category: A Study of the U.S. Pharmaceutical Industry." *Pharmaco-Economics* 7(2): 152–69.

Dranove, D. 1998. "Is There an Underinvestment in R&D about Prevention?" *Journal of Health Economics* 17(1): 117–27.

"Effects of Hypoglycemic Agents on Vascular Complications in Patients with Adult-Onset Diabetes. VIII. Evaluation of Insulin Therapy." 1982. *Diabetes* 31(supplement 5): 1–78.

Estacio, R. O., and others. 1998. "The Effect of Nisoldipine as Compared with Enalapril on Cardiovascular Outcomes in Patients with Non-Insulin-Dependent Diabetes and Hypertension." *New England Journal of Medicine* 338(10): 645–52.

FDA Consumer Website. 1990. http://www.fda.gov/opacom/morechoices/fdaconsumer.html (May), 10.

"The Fifth Report of the Joint National Committee on the Detection, Evaluation, and Treatment of High Blood Pressure (JNCV)." 1993. *Archives of Internal Medicine* 153:154–83.

Formicola, A., R. Gottsegan, and J. Hay. 1981. "Commentary on 'Periodontal Disease: Assessing the Effectiveness and Costs of the Keyes Technique.'" In *Implications of Cost-Effectiveness Analysis of Medical Technology.* Washington, D.C.: Office of Technology Assessment, U.S. Congress.

Fountzilas, G., and others. 1997. "Paclitaxel and Carboplatin in Recurrent and Metastatic Head and Neck Cancer: A Phase II Study." *Seminars in Oncology* 24(1, supplement 2): S2-65-67.

Frick, M. H., and others. 1987. "Helsinki Heart Study: Primary Prevention Trial with Gemfibrozil in Middle-Aged Men with Dyslipidemia: Safety of Treatment, Changes in Risk Factors and Incidence of Coronary Heart Disease." *New England Journal of Medicine* 317: 1237–45.

Furberg, C. D., and B. M. Psaty. 1995. "Dose-Related Increase in Mortality in Patients with Coronary Heart Disease." *Circulation* 92(5): 1326–31.

Ghadirian, P., and others. 1997. "Nutritional Factors and Colon Carcinoma." *Cancer* 80: 858–64.

Gotto, A., for the AFCAPS/TEXCAPS Study Group. 1997. "The AFCAPS/TEXCAPS Study. Abstract." Paper presented to the American Heart Association 70th Annual Meeting, Orlando, Fla.

Grabowski, Henry, and John Vernon. 1998. "Effective Patent Life in Pharmaceuticals." *International Journal of Technology Management* (in press).

Grimm, R. H., Jr. 1989. "Epidemiological and Cost Implications of Antihypertensive Treatment for the Prevention of Cardiovascular Disease." *Journal of Human Hypertension* 3(supplement 2): 55–61.

Grobbee, D. E., and A. W. Hoes. 1995. "Non-Potassium-Sparing Diuretics and Risk of Sudden Cardiac Death." *Journal of Hypertension* 13(12, part 2): 1539–45.

Hay, Joel, and others. 1998. "Health Policy Implications of Extending Marketing Exclusivity for Taxol®." University of Southern California, Los Angeles.

Hortobagyi, G. N., and others. 1997. "Combination Chemotherapy with Paclitaxel and Doxorubicin for Metastatic Breast Cancer." *Seminars in Oncology* 24 (4, supplement 11): S11-13–19.

Kinlay, S., and P. Ganz. 1997. "Role of Endothelial Dysfunction in Coronary Artery Disease and Implications for Therapy." *American Journal of Cardiology* 80(9A): 111–61.

Lipid Research Clinics Program. 1984a. "The Lipid Research Clinics Coronary Primary Prevention Trials Results. I. Reduction in Incidence of Coronary Heart Disease." *Journal of the American Medical Association* 251: 351–64.

———. 1984b. "The Lipid Research Clinical Coronary Primary Prevention Trials Results. II. The Relationship of Reduction in Incidence of Coronary Heart Disease to Cholesterol-Lowering." *Journal of the American Medical Association* 251: 365–74.

Loesche, W. J., and others. 1996. "The Non-Surgical Treatment of Periodontal Patients." *Oral Medicine, Oral Surgery, Oral Pathology* 81: 533–43.

Mark, E. J., and others. 1997. "Fatal Pulmonary Hypertension Associated with Short-Term Use of Fenfluramine and Phentermine." *New England Journal of Medicine* 337(9): 602–06.

Marshall, B. J., and J. R. Warren. 1984. "Unidentified Curved Bacilli in the Stomach of Patients with Gastritis and Peptic Ulceration." *Lancet* (8390): 1311–15.

Max, P. 1997. "Report of National Economic Research Associates, Inc." Washington, D.C.: National Economic Research Associates.

McGuire, W. P., and others. 1996. "Cyclophosphamide and Cisplatin versus Paclitaxel and Cisplatin: A Phase III Randomized Trial in Patients with Suboptimal Stage III/IV Ovarian Cancer (from the Gynecologic Oncology Group)." *Seminars in Oncology* 23(5, supplement 12). 40–47.

Medical Research Council Working Party. 1992. "Medical Research Council Trial of Treatment of Hypertension in Older Adults: Principal Results." *BMJ* 4(6824): 405–12.

Meerpohl, H. G., and others. 1997. "Paclitaxel Combined with Carboplatin in the First Line of Treatment of Advanced Ovarian Cancer: A Phase I Trial." *Seminars in Oncology* 24(1, supplement 2): S17–22.

"National Ambulatory Medical Care Survey, 1995." 1996. Hyattsville, Md.: National Center for Health Statistics.

National Center for Health Statistics. 1994. "Current Estimates from the National Health Interview Survey, 1993." Vital and Health Statistics, series 10, no. 190.

Neil, G. A. 1997. "Do Ulcers Burn out or Burn on? Managing Duodenal Ulcer Diathesis in the *Helicobacter pylori* Era: Ad Hoc Committee on FDA-Related Matters." *American Journal of Gastroenterology* 92: 387–93.

NORDIL Group. 1993. "The Nordic Diltiazem Study (NORDIL): A Prospective Intervention Trial of Calcium Antagonist Therapy in Hypertension." *Blood Pressure* 2(4): 314–21.

Pharmaceutical Information Associates. 1997. "Focus on Peptic Ulcer Disease." Medical Sciences Bulletin. http://pharminfo.com/pubs/msb/peptic.html

Pharmaceutical Research and Manufacturers of America. 1996. Based on data from PhRMA Annual Survey and data from Compustat, as published in *Business Week*, "R&D Scoreboard" (July). http://www.phrma.org/facts/phfacts/index.html

————. 1997. *Facts and Figures* (August). http://www.phrma.org/facts/phfacts/9fl97a. html

Physicians' Health Study Research Group, Steering Committee. 1989. "Final Report on the Aspirin Component of the Ongoing Physicians' Health Study." *New England Journal of Medicine* 321: 129–35.

Pitt, B., and others. 1995. "Pravastatin Limitation of Atherosclerosis in the Coronary Arteries (PLAC-I): Reduction in Atherosclerosis Progression and Clinical Events." *Journal of the American College of Cardiology* 26: 1133–39.

Reder, Dan. 1997. "Cardiovascular Disease: Current Understanding." Paper presented to the Association for Pharmacoeconomics and Outcomes Research Lipid Conference, Orlando, Fla.

Rimm, E. B., and others. 1993. "Vitamin E Consumption and the Risk of Coronary Heart Disease in Men." *New England Journal of Medicine* 328(20): 1450–56.

Rubin, R. J., W. M. Altman, and D. N. Mendelson. 1994. "Health Care Expenditures for People with Diabetes Mellitus, 1992." *Journal of Clinical Endocrinology and Metabolism* 78(4): 809A–809F.

Sacks, F. M., and others. 1996. "The Effect of Pravastatin on Coronary Events after Myocardial Infarction in Patients with Average Cholesterol Levels." *New England Journal of Medicine* 335: 1001–09.

Sano, M., and others. 1997. "A Controlled Trial of Selegiline, Alpha-Tocopherol or Both as Treatment of Alzheimer's Disease: The Alzheimer's Disease Cooperative Study." *New England Journal of Medicine* 336(17): 1216–22.

Saville, M. W., and others. 1995. "Treatment of HIV-Associated Kaposi's Sarcoma with Paclitaxel." *Lancet* 346(8966): 26–28.

Scandinavian Simvastatin Survival Study group. 1994. "Randomized Trial of Cholesterol Lowering in 4444 Patients with Coronary Heart Disease: The Scandinavian Simvastatin Survival Study." *Lancet* 344: 1383–89.

Scherer, F. M., and D. Ross. 1990. *Industrial Market Structure and Economic Performance.* 3d ed. Boston: Houghton Mifflin.

Seltzer, Holbrooke S. 1972. "A Summary of the Conclusions of the Findings and Conclusions of the University Group Diabetes Program (UGDP)." *Diabetes* 21: 976–79.

Shepherd, Jim. 1997. "Lipid Therapy: LDL Lowering Is Not the Only Thing That Matters." Paper presented to the Association for Pharmacoeconomics and Outcomes Research Lipid Conference, Orlando, Fla.

Shepherd, Jim, and others. 1995. "Prevention of Coronary Heart Disease with Pravastatin in Men with Hypercholesterolemia." *New England Journal of Medicine* 333: 1301–07.

Soll, A. H. 1996. "Medical Treatment of Peptic Ulcer Disease: Practice Guidelines." *Journal of the American Medical Association* 275: 622–29.

Sonnenberg. A., and J. E. Everhart. 1997. "Health Impact of Peptic Ulcer in the United States." *American Journal of Gastroenterology* 92(4): 614–20.

Stampfer, M. J., and others. 1993. "Vitamin E Consumption and the Risk of Coronary Heart Disease in Men." *New England Journal of Medicine* 328(20): 1444–49.

Stephens, N. G., and others. 1996. "Randomised Controlled Trial of Vitamin E in Patients with Coronary Disease: Cambridge Heart Antioxidant Study (CHAOS)." *Lancet* 347(9004): 781–86.

Testa, M. A., and others. 1993. "Quality of Life and Antihypertensive Therapy in Men: A Comparison of Captopril with Enalapril." *New England Journal of Medicine* 328(13): 907–13.

Tonkin, Andrew. 1998. "Prevention of Cardiovascular Events and Death with Prevastatin in Patients with Coronary Heart Disease and a Broad Range of Initial Cholesterol Levels." LIPID Study Group. *New England Journal of Medicine* 339(19): 1349–57

United Kingdom Prospective Diabetes Study Group. 1996. "A 9-Year Update of a Randomized Controlled Trial on the Effect of Improved Metabolic Control on Complications in Non-Insulin-Dependent Diabetes Mellitus." *Annals of Internal Medicine* 124(1, part 2): 136–45.

U.S. Congress, Office of Technology Assessment. 1993. "Pharmaceutical R&D: Costs, Risks and Rewards." OTA-H-522. Government Printing Office.

Ward, M., and D. Dranove. 1995. "The Vertical Chain of Medical Research and Development." *Economic Inquiry* 33(1): 70–87.

Wolffenbuttel, B., and T. Haeften. 1995. "Prevention of Complications in Non-Insulin-Dependent Diabetes Mellitus (NIDDM)." *Drugs* 50(2): 263–88.

WOSCOPS Study Group. "Pravastatin Event Reduction Analysis." *Circulation* (in press).

Wysowski, D. K., and T. P. Gross. 1990. "Deaths due to Accidents and Violence in Two Recent Trials in Cholesterol-Lowering Drugs." *Archives of Internal Medicine* 150: 2169–72.

Comments on
Chapter 5

COMMENT BY
Thomas W. Croghan

CHAPTER 5 SUGGESTS that patent laws, which increase incentives to create new drugs, do not adequately provide for expanded, more efficient uses of existing pharmaceutical technologies. The assumption underlying this interesting work is that society needs to expand its understanding of access, quality, and cost related to pharmaceutical services. This type of research is extraordinarily useful to health plans and is the reason that many have developed outstanding services research centers of their own.[1] Hay and Yu may also be correct that current incentives make investments in new therapies relatively attractive when compared to expanding our understanding of older, more established technologies, but the evidence presented does not support their inference that the balance between investments in new technology innovation and investments in understanding new or better use of existing technology is suboptimal.

Hay and Yu attempt to support the conclusion that current policy for patent protection does not achieve optimal societal outcomes with anecdotes designed to convince the reader that both pharmaceutical companies and government have failed in their mandate to produce relevant knowledge about the appropriate uses of medicines and that this is at least in part the result of current patent policy. There are, however, alternative explanations for past underproduction of outcomes research regarding the true societal value of pharmaceuticals and other technologies, including the knowledge that existing treatments, no matter how well they might be applied, will not cure many of today's medical conditions, such as cancer, Alzheimer's disease, AIDS, and arthritis. In addition, a strong

1. Roper (1997).

case can be made that there is sufficient incentive for pharmaceutical manufacturers to seek approval for new and improved uses of their current treatments until the time of composition of matter patent expiry. There are four important considerations. First, in contrast to the assertions of the authors, pharmaceutical companies have been leaders in the outcomes research movement, even before health plans and other customer groups became organized and demanded these research results. Second, there are many examples of pharmaceutical companies pursuing new indications for existing products well into the normal product life cycle. Third, FDA regulation regarding dissemination of information not substantiated by "two adequate and well-controlled studies," the current standard for promotional claims made by pharmaceutical manufacturers, plays a major role in reducing the incentives for outcomes research, but recent reforms may play a substantial role in improving these circumstances. Finally, implementation of the Hay-Yu proposal on use patents may have unintended consequences opposite to those they hypothesize.

Outcomes research in diabetes, much maligned in chapter 5, represents an example of the difficulty of conducting pharmaceutical research and how the scientific process of replication and comment serves society in answering difficult treatment questions. For example, the effects of treatment on cardiovascular mortality in type II diabetes mellitus has been an area of controversy for more than three decades. The findings of the University Group Diabetes Program were first released in 1970 after eight and one-half years of study and suggested that cardiovascular mortality for patients taking tolbutamide was increased by two and one-half times the rate for patients treated with diet alone.[2] Total mortality was not, however, increased. The results of the study were extensively criticized, the criticisms were rebutted, and new studies were initiated.[3] And although tolbutamide continues to have a black box warning on its label, most experts agree that lowering blood glucose in patients with type II diabetes will result in improved morbidity and mortality overall and that oral hypoglycemics have an appropriate and important role in management.[4]

In the meantime, pharmaceutical companies have sponsored important research with the goal of improving treatment of type II diabetes, and specifically with regard to cardiovascular outcomes.[5] Over the years,

2. UGDP (1970).
3. Seltzer (1972); Prout and others (1972).
4. A "black box" is used on a drug's label to highlight specific warnings regarding its use. This space is generally reserved to list the most severe adverse reactions associated with the drug.
5. Hayward and others (1997).

the pharmaceutical industry has also taken a leadership role in determining new uses for its existing products and funding very large outcomes research projects. As the authors point out, the industry has funded large studies of cholesterol reduction in cardiovascular mortality. Pharmaceutical companies have also funded large studies of ACE inhibitors in mortality and quality of life in congestive heart failure and the GUSTO studies of thrombolysis and heart attack.[6] Indeed, in many areas of cardiovascular medicine, large outcomes studies are a requirement for formulary inclusion. In addition, major producers of H2 antagonists sought approval for gastroesophageal reflux disease even as patent expiry loomed for several of their products. These and other examples suggest that the industry has the necessary incentive to sustain active research agendas that include diverse and relevant outcomes, even at times when government funding for agencies such as the Agency for Health Care Policy and Research has declined.

Even if we agree that we could improve on the incentives a pharmaceutical company faces with regard to its outcomes research agenda, I find the use-patent solution naive. The concept of use patents is well known and clearly specified in current legal process. They are used to provide a period of market exclusivity beyond that provided by composition of matter patents and work well when the use of the drug is restricted to a single major use. For example, if the composition of matter patent, which would normally include the projected uses of the new drug, had expired and these original intended uses had not worked, then the company could secure a use patent for a second use, test the idea, and if it works, enjoy a period of market exclusivity. Because this protection exists, companies maintain "files" of all newly synthesized chemical entities, and the chemicals are routinely tested for new uses, occasionally with remarkable success, such as AZT treatment of AIDS.

Hay and Yu demonstrate a fundamental lack of understanding of patent law in their proposal. Indeed, implementation of their proposal would require reconstruction of the statutes. In order to obtain a use patent, the proposed use must be both novel and nonobvious. The example of vitamin E use for prevention of heart disease is neither new nor nonobvious given our current knowledge. Therefore, what Hay and Yu are actually proposing is a system of data exclusivity and compulsory license granted by regulatory authorities. This compulsory license could

---

6. GUSTO, for "Global Use of Streptokinase and TPA in Occlusion," represents a series of studies on the use of appropriate pharmacology for treatment of heart attack. See, for example, the recent review by Califf (1997).

have an extraordinary effect on new drug development because it would not take into account the risk assumed by the original manufacturer for creation and development of the new chemical entity. It seems unlikely, based on work reported elsewhere in this volume, that society would achieve an optimal outcome under these circumstances. Firms would face increased development expenses and a reduction in the probability of recouping investment.

There is a second potential effect on new drug development that is not adequately explored by the authors. Suppose manufacturers faced the possibility that the composition of matter patent would be superseded by a subsequent use patent? The obvious response would be to disclose any and all potential uses of new chemical entities. Under this scenario, the original discoverers of AZT would probably have disclosed its potential use in viral infections and other diseases, and we would not have had AZT treatment for AIDS, an outcome of tragic proportion.

Finally, administration of the patent seems likely to be an extraordinary task. The proposed hierarchical patent structure would require regulatory administration of an essentially legal concept, something for which regulators are not prepared. The level of evidence required to justify use patent protection would be difficult if not impossible to define. Outcomes studies of the type under consideration require introduction of usual care, and in many cases this has effects on the internal validity of the study. Setting the level of evidence too high, as in the current interpretation of the regulations for determination of effectiveness, would have a dampening effect on outcomes research, whereas setting this level too low could create an essential deficit in the supply of patent attorneys necessary to litigate the outcome related to conflicting studies. Finally, enforcement would just not be workable as patent-holders would not realistically sue infringing physicians and patients even if the infringement could be identified. In the end, I find this chapter unsatisfying, its assumptions uninformed, and its prescription naive.

COMMENT BY
Patricia M. Danzon

I N "DRUG PATENTS and Prices: Can We Achieve Better Outcomes?" Joel Hay and Winnie Yu make the important point that the current patent system may entail serious bias in incentives for innovation because some investments are patentable and others are not. Specifically, the authors argue that the current system leaves an underproduction of knowledge regarding relative benefits and costs of alternative treatments, particularly for older or natural products for which product patents cannot be obtained. They therefore propose a system of use patents. While agreeing that there is a problem, I think that their proposed cure may be significantly worse than the disease, for several reasons.

First, they overstate the problem of patenting forms or uses of existing products. For example, special forms of vitamins are patentable and significant research is already under way to demonstrate effects of these vitamins.

Second, they implicitly assume that only randomized controlled trials (RCTs) convey any information and that RCTs convey perfect information. More realistically, information about the effects of new technologies accumulates from actual use as well as RCTs and ultimately remains probabilistic, particularly at the individual patient level. An RCT provides evidence for a specific population under highly controlled, usually unrealistic clinical conditions. By contrast, a retrospective or epidemiological study based on actual use and patient outcomes has greater risk of being biased by unobserved patient and provider heterogeneity but has less risk of being biased by unrealistic treatment protocols and unrepresentative patient characteristics.

Third, even if retrospective studies convey less useful information than RCTs, retrospective studies also cost vastly less. The only costs of a retrospective study are computing costs and some time of low-paid economists. The costs of an RCT, as would presumably be required to obtain a use patent, are potentially huge. They include:

1. Clinical costs of actually conducting the trial, which includes clinician time and patient treatment costs.

2. Possible risks to patients as investigators seek to undertake trials with potentially patentable results (unless the FDA strictly regulates which trials can be undertaken, in which case regulatory costs would partially replace patient risk costs).

3. Forgone health benefits due to delay in treatment, if payers routinely require such trials before paying for new technologies, many of which are beneficial.

4. Litigation costs of defining the margins of a use patent. Conflict could arise at several margins, including defining patient subgroups and size of effects. For example, if you showed that drug A reduces mortality for a given population by 10 percent, but I show that for a population

subgroup it reduces mortality by 20 percent, does my patent trump yours? Does improvement in quality of life trump a more specific but more statistically significant effect on a narrower dimension of clinical outcome?

5. Excessive research and development investments in the race to capture the monopoly profits inherent in patents.

6. Deadweight loss from suboptimal use of patented products, if patents permit prices to rise above marginal cost.

Deadweight losses due to pricing above marginal cost are potentially more serious than with a standard product patent because a use patent would often be superimposed on the product patent. It is well known that two-tier monopoly generates greater deadweight loss than single-tier monopoly—indeed, eliminating the excess inefficiency of two-tier monopoly is often a motive for vertical integration. Although it is likely that a use patent would be held by the owner of the product patent in order to eliminate this excess inefficiency of two-tier monopoly as well as because of the information advantages, nevertheless this would not always be the case. Moreover, it seems likely that the superimposing conflicting patents would often be the practical solution to conflicting margins of use patents noted in item 4 above, in which case layering of multiple, separately owned patents could occur. It is conceivable that a system of competitive entry to capture use patents could reduce the mean and increase the variance of expected revenues for product patents, such that investment in developing new products would be reduced as a result of the use-patent system.

In addition, Hay and Yu seriously underestimate the enforcement problems, particularly in the case of nonprescription products that have multiple uses. For example, if vitamin E is shown to reduce risk of heart disease but is also believed to have other health benefits, how can consumers' purpose in buying the over-the-counter product be determined? What if they hope that it will have multiple benefits, only some of which are covered by use patents? Similar problems arise if a use patent could exist for a product that is desired for its own sake. For example, if someone demonstrates and obtains a use patent for vitamin C to prevent colds, must I pay a use tax to the patent-holder every time I eat an orange? Only in winter? More appropriately, the tax should be paid only on the additional oranges I eat because of the additional information provided by the holder of the use patent. Determining the appropriate use tax on such multi-use, nonprescription products clearly creates prohibitive information problems.

Finally, even if use patents could be enforced on proof of benefits of prescription products and procedures, that still leaves serious bias in financial incentives for investment in health-related information more generally. There is still no financial incentive to invest in showing that something is not useful or is positively harmful. There is also no financial incentive to develop information that is intrinsically unpatentable, such as information on the effects, beneficial or harmful, of behavior modification such as exercise, stress reduction, and abstaining from smoking. Since the reach of use patents would be at best limited, such a system might generate a worse skew in resource allocation to health-related information, with a larger share going to demonstrate patentable beneficial effects of new products and even less on unpatentable effects, including harmful products and all behavior modification. Increased funding to the National Institutes of Health (NIH) or to endowed chairs in preventive medicine seem to offer a lower-cost, more neutral approach to the problem of information under-production than the use-patent system proposed here.

COMMENT BY
Henry Grabowski

THE CENTRAL THESIS of Hay and Yu's chapter, "Drug Patents and Prices: Can We Achieve Better Outcomes?," is that there are strong market failures with respect to the production of socially beneficial knowledge for a wide range of currently marketed drugs. In this regard, they point out that firms have little economic incentive to conduct expensive trials for new indications of a drug after its product patents have expired and generic suppliers have entered the market. In particular, it is difficult for the inventor to appropriate the benefits from a use patent in the presence of several competing producers (the well-known "free rider" problem).

They also point out that many drugs are approved for marketing based on surrogate endpoints (for example, changes in blood pressure), although our real interest is in their effect on health outcomes (for example, changes in mortality or the quality of life). Hay and Yu present many case examples to show that little is known about the latter outcomes for large classes of important drug therapies. They also attribute this to a market failure incentive problem associated with the intellectual property rights system.

The novelty of Hay and Yu's essay is primarily in its policy prescriptions. They advocate several steps to improve the enforcement of use patents in order to encourage research on drug outcomes and new indications. Before analyzing their policy proposals, I find it instructive to discuss drug use patents in more detail. Such patents are in fact currently employed by pharmaceutical firms as the primary form of patent protection in some circumstances when a product or composition of matter patent is not possible. One prominent example is AZT, the first breakthrough drug to treat AIDS.

AZT was first synthesized by Dr. Jerome Horowitz of the Detroit Institute for Cancer Research in 1964. However, the drug proved ineffective as a cancer remedy. The compound remained unpatented and in the public domain until the mid-1980s, when Burroughs-Wellcome examined it as a possible AIDS treatment because of its observed activity against retroviruses in mice. When it proved effective against the HIV virus in humans, Burroughs-Wellcome applied for and obtained both a use patent and orphan drug exclusivity rights.[7]

The orphan drug exclusivity for AZT expired in 1994, but its use patent remains in effect until the year 2005.[8] It is the principal form of intellectual property rights for this important drug. In this case, AZT is protected only for its AIDS indication. However, since there are no other approved uses, it effectively protects this compound from market entry by other suppliers. If another drug manufacturer were to discover a new use for AZT, it could apply to the FDA for marketing approval. However, it would have to submit a regular new drug application demonstrating its efficacy in this use based on new clinical trial data.

A few new chemical entries are approved each year with use patents as their primary form of patent protection.[9] As the AZT case illustrates, use patents can work very well when there is only a single approved use for a particular drug. However, these patent rights do not work as well when there are already multiple suppliers for a different use. This is the point of several market failure examples in the Hay-Yu chapter (antibiotic treatment of ulcers, the use of vitamin E to prevent cardiovascular problems, and so on).

7. Emmons and Nimgade (1991).

8. FOI Services (1997).

9. This number may go up in the future as firms use high-throughput screening methods on large libraries of synthesized compounds. Mass ligand screening methods allow firms to evaluate millions of compounds for particular kinds of biological activity. They represent a very large potential productivity advance over traditional screening approaches using whole animal models. See the discussion of these methods in Lehman Brothers (1997).

A use patent currently gives the holder certain property rights. The holder is the only supplier that can advertise the effectiveness of the product for that use. Moreover, the inventing firm can also sue consumers who purchase an alternative product for the protected use. However, the high transactions costs of enforcing such a patent against hundreds of thousands of users, and the disinclination on the part of firms to sue their customers, have typically made this an empty property right.

There are some trends currently at work to lower the enforcement costs on use patents. The growth of managed care has made the demand side of the market much more concentrated in nature. Hence, it is now possible to focus enforcement efforts on the large institutional payors. In addition, virtually all the nation's pharmacies have been computerized to handle the claims processing of prescriptions on line.[10] Eventually, experts also expect that the physician's prescriptions will be sent to pharmacies through computer networks.

One interesting aspect of Hay and Yu's proposal is that they would require physicians to specify the intended use of a drug product on their prescriptions. In the new world of computerized prescriptions, this would allow firms to readily target large institutional violators of their use patents. However, I think it is still questionable whether drug firms would sue their managed care customers for purchasing lower-priced generic versions. I think they are unlikely to do so, given that the products at issue would represent only a small fraction of the revenues at stake in the managed care market, and such an action could lead to unfavorable repercussions.

Nevertheless, making physicians specify the intended use of a product on their prescription seems like a worthwhile market experiment that is also desirable on other grounds. It would be interesting to see whether it improves the enforcement of current property rights on use patents. In any event, it could provide some useful information, and I do not think it would do any harm.

However, such expanded use patents are unlikely to help much in the case of over-the-counter products like vitamin E that do not require a doctor's prescription and are not even reimbursed by many health care payors. It would seem that if a product like vitamin E can yield high potential medical benefits through a new use, this is precisely the public goods type of situation for which a government grant from the NIH or Agency for Health Care Policy and Research is appropriate. This would

10. Grabowski and Mullins (1997).

appear to be the most cost-beneficial approach in this particular situation. Government agencies could also explore partnership arrangements with consortiums of managed care organizations to support such studies. An alliance of MCOs might be willing to bear part of the costs since they potentially stand to realize some of the collective economic benefits in this kind of situation.

Although requiring physicians to specify the use of drugs on prescriptions seems worthwhile, I am quite skeptical about the other elements of the Hay-Yu proposal for use patents. In particular, they call for a hierarchical system of use-patent claims. Under their plan, a firm that develops evidence that extends the scope of a product's medical claims through outcome analysis would override any use patents based on narrower claims. This part of their proposal is designed to encourage more post-marketing outcome assessments (so-called phase IV studies).

I believe this aspect of their use-patent proposal is fraught with high social costs relative to the potential social benefits. It would require the FDA to set the evidentiary standards on use claims and would expand the number and scope of FDA regulatory determinations severalfold. Hence, there is the likelihood of increased bureaucratic delays and errors. It could also lead to many unintended costs as a result of firms engaging in strategic behavior to override each other's patents. The use of improvement patents in other circumstances does not provide a very encouraging model to emulate in this situation.[11]

I do not share the authors' view that the lack of outcome studies for many important drugs is basically a failure of the intellectual property rights system. Rather, I think it is more of a reflection of our traditional fee-for-service insurance system, which did not demand that these studies be performed. In the past, there was a strong imperative for providers to embrace newer high-priced technologies in pharmaceuticals (and other medical areas) once regulatory officials certified that they were safe and effective. However, as the health care system has shifted toward managed care and prospective payment systems, these incentives have changed dramatically. As a consequence, outcome studies on new drug products have become an area of tremendous growth for pharmaceutical firms.[12]

One instructive example is the case of the two thrombolytic agents, TPA and streptokinase. The recombinant product TPA has a much higher cost than the older product streptokinase (on the order of $2,200 versus

11. Scotchmer (1996a, 1996b).
12. Sloan and Grabowski (1997).

$270 for each treatment). In the current world of cost consciousness and DRGs (diagnostic related groups), hospital decisionmakers want proof that the higher costs of TPA are more than offset by higher expected benefits. To demonstrate that this was the case, Genentech sponsored the GUSTO clinical trial, a head-to-head randomized clinical trial between TPA and streptokinase that involved 40,000 patients and cost over $65 million. Forty thousand patients were enrolled in this clinical trial in order to demonstrate that there was a statistically significant 1 percent difference in mortality rates between TPA and streptokinase.[13] As expected, the outcome of the GUSTO study and the cost-effectiveness studies based on it have affected TPA's usage by hospitals.

Most outpatient drugs are not yet subject to the same cost-containment pressures as those for inpatient drugs like TPA, but this is the way the world is moving. Managed care entities are currently implementing more restrictive drug formularies.[14] In this new environment, drugs that can demonstrate superior outcome profiles will be able to negotiate better prices and avoid onerous usage restrictions (prior authorization, step therapy protocols, and so on). These developments have produced an explosive growth in outcome studies (both pre- and postmarketing studies) as firms look forward to where the health care system will be in the year 2000 and beyond.

Given current developments in worldwide health care, it is difficult to support the view that there is a pervasive incentive problem on the part of drug firms to perform outcome studies, as Hay and Yu claim. Firms have strong incentives to perform these studies for novel new drug entities with long patent lives if they want them included on the managed care formularies of the future.[15] Of course, many older compounds for which patent rights are short or have already expired may fall through the cracks in terms of both outcome assessments and research on new indications. This is why third-party groups and academic institutions will continue to have a strong role to play in performing new studies, as well as assessing the worth of existing studies.

References

Califf, Robert M. 1997. "The GUSTO Trial and the Open Artery Theory." *European Heart Journal* 18 (supplement F) (December): F2–10.

13. Mark and others (1995)
14. Grabowski (1998).
15. Grabowski and Vernon (1999).

Emmons, Willis, and Ashok Nimgade. 1991. "Burroughs Wellcome and AZT." Case 9-792-004. Harvard Business School.

FOI Services. 1997. *Drugs under Patent.* Gaithersburg, Md.: FOI Services.

Grabowski, Henry. 1998. "The Role of Cost Effectiveness Studies in Managed Care Decisions." *Pharmacoeconomics* 14 (supplement 1): 15–24.

Grabowski, Henry, and C. Daniel Mullins. 1997. "Pharmacy Benefit Management, Cost-Effectiveness Analyses, and Drug Formulary Decisions." *Social Science and Medicine* 45(4) (August): 535–44.

Grabowski, Henry, and John Vernon. 1999. "Effective Patent Life in Pharmaceuticals." *International Journal of Technology Management* (in press).

Hayward, R. A., and others. 1997. "Starting Insulin Therapy in Patients with Type 2 Diabetes: Effectiveness, Complications, and Resource Utilization." *Journal of the American Medical Association* 278: 1663–69.

Mark, E. J., and others. 1997. "Fatal Pulmonary Hypertension Associated with Short-Term Use of Fenfluramine and Phentermine." *New England Journal of Medicine* 337(9): 602–06.

Prout, Thaddeus E., and others. 1972. "The UGDP Controversy: Clinical Trials versus Clinical Implications." *Diabetes* 21: 1035–40.

Scotchmer, Susan, 1996a. "Protecting Early Innovators: Should Second-Generation Products Be Patentable?" *RAND Journal of Economics* 27(2) (Summer): 322–31.

———. 1996b. "Patents as an Incentive System." In *Economics in a Changing World,* edited by B. Allen. Vol. 2. New York: St. Martin's Press.

Seltzer, Holbrooke S. 1972. "A Summary of the Conclusions of the Findings and Conclusions of the University Group Diabetes Program (UGDP)." *Diabetes* 21: 976–79.

Sloan, Frank, and Henry Grabowski, eds. 1997. *The Impact of Cost Effectiveness on Public and Private Policies on Health Care: An International Perspective. Introduction and Overview.* Special issue of *Social Science and Medicine* 45(4) (August): 505–10.

"UGDP: A Study of the Effects of Oral Hypoglycemic Agents on Vascular Complications in Patients with Adult-Onset Diabetes." 1970. *Diabetes* 19 (supplement 2): 747–830.

6

Medical Care Costs, Benefits, and Effects: Conceptual Issues for Measuring Price Changes

Mark V. Pauly

IN AN EVER changing world, neither prices nor products remain stable. The phenomenon of change prevails everywhere in modern economics, but there are few sectors where it is more pervasive but less transparent than in the medical care sector. In addition to the usual pattern of changing input prices and changing prices for alternative products, medical care is the example par excellence of changing products and changing technology. Especially in the last decade, changes in product have been matched by an accelerated pace of changes in insurance arrangements, illness types, patient expectations, and consumer tastes.

In the midst of this change, spending on medical services continues to rise, although at lower rates recently than previously. It would be of great benefit if we could determine how much of this increased spending—in the past, in the present, or (probably) in the future—represents price increases and how much of it represents changes in quality or quantity.

There has been a large increase in interest in, and some improvement in results of, techniques to compare the spending or costs of medical services with their outcomes. Cost-effectiveness and cost-benefit analysis of medical services is a growth industry. In this chapter I categorize these techniques and analyze their suitability for the construction of a price index for medical care that is valid from the viewpoint of welfare economics. I argue that there are a number of different measures that might be somewhat useful, depending in part on what the desired framework for the analysis of price change is. My most novel conclusion, however, is that one useful measure of overall medical care price change, possible (with sufficient research effort) and desirable, is the change in consumer willingness to pay for insured medical services covered by a managed care insurance plan. This measure, I argue, could form the basis of a conceptually valid and practically useful "quality deflator" of expenditures for medical care and would be a desirable adjunct or alternative to measures such as quality-adjusted life-years (QALYs) and other physical or utility-based measures derived from cost-effectiveness analysis. I will also argue that consideration of the choice between these two types of measures throws useful analytic light on both.

The Price of What?

More than 80 percent of medical care spending in the United States is covered by health insurance, public or private. Most of this insurance now contains some elements of managed care. These two considerations imply that the relevant measure of quality is *insured* quality, not quality as experienced by someone paying out of pocket. The two notions are different because the relevant impact of quality accompanying an expenditure change, the effect on an insured person's utility or well-being, is an effect that can differ from that of technically identical quality and the same expenditure change on the utility of an uninsured person.

Concretely, this means that the appropriate measure of quality change is the incremental willingness to pay the premium for a managed care plan that supplies the new service (compared to the premium for an otherwise identical plan that does not). This observation suggests a daring possibility: rejuvenate and modify a suggestion made decades ago by Melvin Reder. Define the price of medical care as the premium for insurance, but use the managed care insurance premium and adjust the premium for quality change using willingness-to-pay techniques.[1] The objections raised at the time to Reder's measures are now less valid. Managed care plans vary much less in coverage than indemnity plans and usually have minimal cost sharing. The development of willingness-to-pay techniques provides a vehicle for quality adjustment that was not available when Reder wrote.

Americans do not consume medical services; they buy insured medical care. Moreover, they pay for the great bulk of this medical care not by

1. Reder (1969).

paying explicit premiums but by accepting lower wages, a behavior not incorporated into the current medical CPI. It therefore follows that a proper and superior measure of value is the value of insured medical care. For a given batch of medical services, this value will generally differ from their value if paid for at the point of use for two reasons: (1) for risk-averse consumers, insurance is valuable; (2) insurance loosens the short-term budget constraint that may limit willingness to pay.[2] These reasons both imply that the proper measure of value to use to deflate total spending will be one that takes into account the insured nature of the great bulk of medical consumption.

Some Preliminary Considerations

We first need to specify what a price index for a particular product or set of products is supposed to measure. A price index should tell us how much better or worse off price changes make a particular set of consumers. Slightly more formally, if the expenditure on a particular good or basket of goods changes, a price index measures the amount of additional income needed to be provided to the consumer (for price increases) or taken away from the consumer (for price decreases) to leave him or her as well off as before a change. Obviously, if the quality and quantity of the product or products being evaluated do not change, the price index is just the percentage change in total spending. In the cases I will be considering here, quantities will not change but quality will. It is obvious that when quality changes, the measure of the change in total expenditure needs to be adjusted to account for the quality change. For example, if spending increased but quality increased as well, an increase in income equal to the change in spending would overcompensate the consumer. Clearly the measure of quality change must be made commensurate with the change in spending to adjust a price index for change in quality.

One reason why an improved price index for medical services in particular is an issue is precisely because there are strong reasons to believe that the quality of those services has been changing over time. The fact of technological change in medical goods and services is undeniable, and contemporaneous improvements in survival hint (though they do not prove) that this quality change may be having some positive

2. Gafni (1991).

impact on health. Another reason for seeking an improved index is that, because of the presence of both public health insurance and tax-subsidized private health insurance, there is no strong basis for expecting consumers to equate marginal values to marginal prices for medical services. (For medical insurance, it may be another story.) Hence, an index independent of direct market price signals may be required.

There has been substantial research devoted to measuring the benefits and outcomes from new medical technologies. Those effects ought ideally to include (but not be limited to) effects on mortality, effects on morbidity, effects on risk reduction or reassurance, and effects on other values (such as reproduction or appearance). The analytical problem is therefore twofold: health is affected by factors other than the quantity and quality of medical care; and medical care is demanded for more reasons than health. For both of these reasons, health measures alone are sure to be inadequate as satisfactory quality measures for medical care.

Costs, Benefits, Effectiveness, and Quality Adjustment

There are, broadly speaking, two different types of techniques that have been developed and used to analyze the consequences of specific costly medical care interventions, including (especially) newly developed interventions: cost-effectiveness analysis and cost-benefit analysis. Cost-effectiveness analysis measures some of the consequences of an intervention in monetary terms and some in nonmonetary terms. Cost-benefit analysis converts all impacts into monetary terms. The nonmonetary part of cost-effectiveness analysis can be either a physical measure (such as expected life-years added) or a utility-based measure (such as quality of well-being). There are also some techniques that adjust physical measures using utility-based approaches (some versions of quality-adjusted life-years). The version of cost-benefit analysis most consistent with welfare economics converts all effects of an intervention, both resources used and health and other outcomes, into money using willingness-to-pay (or be paid) measures.

Either of these analytical techniques could furnish the basis of quality adjustment of change in total expenditure. For instance, consider a change in technology that only improves survival (for example, by preventing or curing a fatal illness of short duration). The quality change could be measured either by the added life-years or by the monetary value consumers would attach to coverage of the survival-improving intervention by their HMO. In what follows, I will try to explain and contrast these alternative approaches to quality measurement.

Modeling Technical Change

The special issues of quality change for medical insurance arise because medical technology changes, not because insurance plans add more previously invented quality to their plans but because insurance itself causes patients as buyers to demand levels of quality without properly considering their cost. How can we define this kind of technological change in this setting? A characterization suggested by James Baumgardner provides a way of thinking about these issues. In figure 6-1, the variable measured along the horizontal axis represents the quantity of real medical services, and the demand curves D_i (of which three are drawn) represent either demand curves for care or money marginal valuation schedules, conditional on the person's state of health or illness. Thus D_S is the marginal valuation schedule for a person with a severe illness, D_M is the curve for a person with a mild illness, and D_I is the curve for an illness of intermediate severity. The unit price of care that the insurance plan must reimburse is $\$P$, but the user price paid by the insured is the (much) lower copayment $\$C$.

Baumgardner represents the limits to technology by a boundary such as the line B_0. Beyond this point, medical care that will improve health and other aspects of well-being cannot be supplied, no matter how high the marginal valuation. (For instance, under current technology, metastasized ovarian cancer cannot be cured.) An improvement in technology is then represented by a shift in B, say, from B_0 to B_1. It can be seen that the net change in overall welfare from improved insured quality may be either positive or negative. For persons with the severe illness, the change in the diagram is positive: the additional consumers' surplus is area ABCD. Technical change produces negative consumers' surplus (welfare loss) in the case of the mild illness, indicated by area DCEF. In the case of the intermediate illness, as drawn, the effects cancel out (area EHJ equals area JDG). The overall expected or average effect depends on the probabilities of each severity as well as the magnitudes of gains or losses. It is the evaluation of such "boundary shifting" technology that is the complex but key piece of information needed to adjust the change over time in managed care premiums for quality improvement.

In contrast, technology that lowered cost in a situation in which the level of outcome was not changed would be entirely embodied in the

Figure 6-1. *Technical Change under Health Insurance*

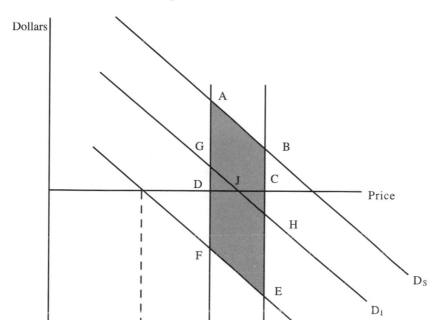

Source: Author's calculations.

premium change. For example, suppose there was a target level of health to be achieved for people with some illness (for example, functional status for patients with depression, blood pressure control for hypertension) and new technology allowed that goal to be achieved in a less costly fashion. Then a managed care plan whose objective it was to meet the goal (neither exceeding it nor falling short) would see its costs and its break-even premium decline by the amount of cost saving.[3]

The illness-state probabilities will change little over time. In that sense the managed care insurance basket will contain the same items ("treatment of a mild illness," "treatment of a severe illness," and so on), so the usual index number weighting problems can be avoided. However, the serious challenge will be measuring the amount and, most important, the *value* of quality change.

3. Berndt and others (1996).

Finally, note that under Baumgardner's view of technology, this value of quality change will tend to vary over "units" of output (for example, health) precisely because the demand curves display diminishing marginal values. This diminishing marginal valuation will hold even if quality changes per time period are identical in terms of their effects on added years of survival or other physical measures.

Lay of the Land

As noted above, a number of different methods for measuring improved outcomes for medical services have been developed. They generally fall into three broad areas: (1) unidimensional health measures, like life expectancy; (2) multidimensional physical or utility-based health measures, such as quality-adjusted life-years, which account for morbidity in life expectancy–based measures by changing the scale by which additional years of life are measured; and (3) summary measures of willingness to pay (contingent valuation) for the full spectrum of changes associated with new technology.

Since the key issue in adjusting price changes for quality variations is developing a measure of quality, it seems natural to consider the measures of effectiveness already constructed for program evaluation in health care. Cost-effectiveness analysis, most commonly applied to pharmaceuticals but also used for other interventions, has been under continuous development and used in health policy analysis for the past fifteen years or so.[4] This technique has largely been elaborated by noneconomists.

The alternative to the nonmonetary outcome measures used in cost-effectiveness analysis is to measure the outcome directly in monetary value terms, and the history of this technique shows more variation. There was a burst of interest in using the human capital approach for benefits measurement more than twenty years ago, but then it died out in most circles for both theoretical and policy reasons. However, within the past five years there has been a rekindling of interest in benefits measurement in the form of direct willingness-to-pay measures established using contingent valuation techniques.[5] These techniques elicit how much the person would be willing to pay for the improvement in question. Before I consider the specific application of any of these measures for purposes

4. Gold and others (1996).
5. Cummings, Brookshire, and Schulze (1986).

of price index measurement, it may be worthwhile to discuss their conceptual foundations in the program analysis context.

Let us begin with the simplest nonmonetary measure of health outcome, life expectancy (or added life-years). It is clear that more years of life will generally be preferred to less, at least as long as the quality of life is above some very minimal level. If there is no other difference (including net cost) between two programs, the one offering longer life expectancy is to be preferred. Moreover, if the program budget is fixed, allocating it among programs based on money costs per year of life added will generally lead to a superior outcome. Without a fixed budget, however, rational resource allocation requires that someone, explicitly or implicitly, decides what extra years of life are worth in money or opportunity cost terms in order to determine the size of the budget. Valuation in commensurate terms is unavoidable.[6]

Suppose then that some boundary shift affects only survival. How would one use this information to determine how much of a managed care insurance plan's premium change was a pure price change under the willingness-to-pay approach? What is required to convert an increment in survival into a monetary measure (for an increase in survival) is an estimate of the maximum amount a buyer would be willing to pay for another year of survival, adjusted for the risk-related aspects of the intervention.

Many medical interventions do more than add to survival (and many do not even do that). Thus there needs to be some method to combine multiple *dimensions* of consequences into a single measure of effect. Virtually by definition, an intervention that improves well-being without increasing survival increases the quality of life. There are many techniques for measuring the quality of life, ranging from asking respondents to score descriptions of life with various maladies on a scale or thermometer to more sophisticated approaches that transform quality into quantity (and back again) by asking respondents about hypothetical trade-offs they would make, then using responses to sketch out a hypothetical (and fairly restrictive) utility function. (Despite the size and growth of the quality-of-life measurement industry, there are almost no tests of the validity of these hypothetical trade-offs based on actual health care behavior: seeing whether people actually would choose an option with a higher alleged quality of life.) Here again, to make a resource

6. Phelps and Mushlin (1991).

allocation decision when the budget is not fixed, someone, somehow, must assign a money value to additional quality adjusted life-years for some population. Likewise, to use the QALY measure for a price index, monetary values must be attached.

Why Is This Important?

It is important to get as accurate a measure as possible of quality for medical treatments in order to be able to construct an acceptable price index because, at least according to conventional health economics wisdom, it is the change in medical services quality or technology, not increases in quantities of unchanging homogeneous services or increases in their prices, that has been by far the most important determinant of real (general inflation adjusted) growth in medical services spending for the last thirty years.[7] Traditional government statistics from the government's Health Care Financing Administration that decompose the growth in total spending into "prices" and "other things" invariably find that neither CPI-type price indexes nor demographic demand shifters explain the bulk of spending growth.[8] Mild-mannered government statisticians usually label this residual "volume and intensity," but economists with tenure are more likely to label it "technological change." The "volume and intensity" increases have come about as new services, new procedures, and new programs were added, even as total hospital days and admissions were dropping and physician encounters per capita held constant.

In which way then will a new technology, which I will label a "program," bias price index measures? The answer, it is clear, depends on the *value* of the new program. To take the benchmark case first (and a situation that would prevail in ordinary markets), if spending were to increase on a basket of medical goods and services because of a new type of program but the value of the new program just equaled the increase in spending, welfare would not increase. It would therefore be correct to say that prices rose as rapidly as spending, so that "real medical consumption" remained the same. However, virtually the entire analysis of American health care policy in the last thirty years has been based on the view that the market did not function like ordinary markets. Often, it was felt, the new technology was likely to be worth less than its opportunity costs. Whether the cause was health insurance, consumer ignorance and

7. Fuchs (1996).
8. Levit and others (1996).

consequent demand inducement, or a postulated "technological imperative," the effect was hypothesized to be the same: the U.S. medical care
sector has fostered some changes in technology whose value has fallen far
short of their cost.[9]

The main problem with contingent valuation approaches to measuring
this value is not so much theoretical as it is practical. Can we obtain
contingent valuation methods with some claim to validity? Although
considerably more effort has been put into effectiveness measures, in this
decade there are a number of willingness-to-pay studies for medical
services that have been published and that have face validity.[10]

There has actually been a larger body of work on contingent valuation
for environmental changes.[11] This work has been criticized as imprecise
because it asks people about public goods, for which they would never
have to pay explicitly.[12] In contrast, most medical services are private
goods, for which people must pay directly or through private insurance.
Nevertheless, some of the techniques for contingent valuation studies of
environmental change (such as the use of "closed-ended" questions)
have been found useful for medical services, and decision supports have
been found to be helpful.

These methods have, however, not generally been used to value large-
scale system changes in health care. Their strength is their ability to keep
the focus on the initial details of specific interventions. To implement
them in the price index context, however, it would be necessary to describe in detail all the changes in technology in a given time period and
ask for an aggregate willingness to pay for the batch. This may prove
difficult.

An alternative hybrid approach is to measure each year's benefits in
physical or utility terms, aggregate those measures, and then monetize
the value. The proper monetization of a physical measure is based on the
willingness to pay for marginal increments in that measure. Where might
such monetization come from, and how useful will the results be?

In most cost-effectiveness studies, determination of the precise money
value of a QALY has not been important. As long as there is no artificial

9. Baumgardner (1991); Goddeeris (1984).

10. Appel and others (1990); Donaldson and Shackley (1997); Eastaugh (1991); Johannesson
(1992); Johannesson, Johnsson, and Borquist (1991); Johannesson and Weinstein (1993); Kartman, Andersson, and Johannesson (1996); Lindhlom, Rosen, and Hellsten (1994); O'Brien and
others (1998); Ramsey and others (1997); Ryan, Ratcliffe, and Tucker (1997); Zelthraseus and
others (1997).

11. Cummings, Brookshire, and Schulze (1986).

12. Diamond and Hausman (1994).

limit on the budget, once the cost and the QALYs from a program have been measured, it is only necessary to determine that the value per QALY is large enough that the benefit per QALY exceeds the cost per QALY. For a price index, however, it is not enough to determine whether the value exceeds some threshold.

Generally speaking, the threshold value per QALY is usually said to be in the range of $25,000–50,000—a suggestion first made in the 1980s. Surprisingly, this value is still used in 1997, without adjustment for fifteen years of economywide inflation.[13] More seriously, there is no obvious source to validate these measures. Experts are asked to pick a number for the value on which they cannot possibly be an expert, a league table of projects ranked by dollars per QALY is used to indicate that projects subjectively judged (on other unspecified grounds) are reasonable, or politicians are asked what they think. Some European economists have in fact endorsed such an extra-welfarist approach to valuation.[14] Whatever their merits in program planning, it would appear to be mildly preposterous to use political valuations to measure quality in a consumer price index. The advantage of the consensus method then is not its credibility. Rather, for the advocate it is its transparency: all beneficial effects are boiled down to QALYs, and then different money values can be proposed. For the cynic, its advantage is that it reserves for experts the final decisionmaking power but disguises the arbitrary nature of the valuation process in a smokescreen of health outcome measurement. It obscures the fact that multiplying precisely and objectively measured QALYs by a subjective arbitrary value yields only a subjectively determined product as the final measure.

There is an alternative approach to the expert consensus method: use money values of health inferred from market behavior that affects or is affected by mortality or morbidity. For the reasons discussed above, behavior in the market for medical services has not been thought to be reliable as a basis for value. Instead, virtually all of the estimates we have are from the labor or real estate markets, where people who avoid dangerous jobs or polluted neighborhoods pay for the privilege. In his summary of this work, Kip Viscusi notes that estimates of the value of life cover a wide range.[15] The central tendency estimates (themselves ranging from $3 million to $7 million) imply for an adult with about forty more years of life expectancy a value per life-year two or three times as large

13. Meltzer (1997); I am indebted to Henry Glick for this latter observation.
14. Sugden and Williams (1978).
15. Viscusi (1993).

as the expert consensus number—and the values from labor market studies are thought to be underestimates of the average value. Moreover, there has been little investigation of whether the labor market–type valuations would also apply to quality-of-life dimensions: whether the valuation of a year of survival, given quality of life, is the same valuation as would be placed on quality of life, given survival.

Your Money or Your Life: What Difference Does the Type of Measure Make?

In principle, a measure of quality change with which to adjust a measure of expenditure change in order to generate a measure of pure price change can be based either on a physical measure or a monetary measure, on "effectiveness" or "benefits." However, the two measures can lead to quite different conclusions in a given empirical situation about what is happening to prices. Here I provide a simplified and hypothetical numerical example to show that the type of measure does matter.

To avoid complexity, consider a new technology whose only health effect is to increase expected survival, but that also necessarily increases total costs and total spending. Other things are going on in this hypothetical economy, however, so we want to partition a given observed increase in total spending to the part attributed to quality improvement and the part attributed to the pure price increase.

Row 1 of table 6-1 shows the amount by which total spending increased in both the previous period and in a number of alternative scenarios for the current period. The previous period increase in spending was $100, as described in column 1. In the initial scenario we examine in column 2, the current period increase is also $100, or a 10 percent increase on a base of $1,000 total spending ($E_o$). How much of this 10 percent is quality change, and how much of it is pure price change?

The second row of the table shows the change in outcome, that is, the number of units of survival ("effect") added as a result of the change in total expenditure; in the benchmark scenario in column 2, the additional survival in the current period is 4 units. How then do we divide the spending change into the component due to quality change and the component due to pure price change? If we use an externally specified money value or willingness-to-pay measure, it is easy to see how to compute the improvement in quality: just multiply the number of units of additional survival by the value of a unit. The table shows two alternative values in rows 6 and 7: $10 per unit and $40 per unit. Using these values,

Table 6-1. *Illustration of Alternative Measures of Quality Change*

Assume E_O = 1,000

	1	2	3	4	5
Δ expenditure	100	100	100	60	100
Δ outcome	5	4	2	3	6
Δ expenditure/					
Δ outcome	20	25	50	20	16.7
Percent Δ expenditure	10	10	10	6	10
Percent Δ quality					
Physical measure	...	8	4	6	12
Value measure					
If $V = 10$	5	4	2	3	6
Value measure					
If $V = 40$	20	16	8	12	24
Percent Δ price					
Physical measure	...	1.9	5.8	0	−1.8
Value measure					
If $V = 10$	4.8	5.8	7.8	2.9	3.8
Value measure					
If $V = 40$	−8.3	−5.2	1.9	−5.4	−11.3

the percentage changes in quality in the current period in the scenario in column 2 are 4 and 16 percent, respectively.

An alternative way to measure quality change uses only physical measures without resort to external values. Even here, however, some monetary weighting of the physical effect will be required in order to convert into an index commensurate with the change in total expenditure. One way of doing so, as indicated in chapter 7, generates a money measure by calculating the marginal cost of adding a unit of survival in the previous period. The data for this calculation are shown in column 1. The cost per unit of survival added (row 3) was $20 in the previous period. Were the cost of adding units of survival to be the same in the current period, this approach would conclude that price did not increase at all in the current period; the percentage increase in quality would equal the percentage increase in expenditure. (Such a case is shown in the scenario in column 4, where the percentage change in price calculated using the "physical measure" approach is indeed shown to be zero.) In the benchmark scenario in column 2, however, this approach would indicate a positive increase in price of about 2 percent (row 8), because the value of the increase in outcome would be estimated to be 4 × 20 = 80, and so "quality" would increase by 8 percent (row 5) while expenditures increased by 10 percent. A measure based on the assumption that the value of a unit is $10 (row 9) would also indicate a positive increase in quality-adjusted price. In contrast, basing the quality index on the assumption that the value of a unit is $40 would lead to the conclusion that quality-adjusted prices actually fell in the scenario of column 2 by more than 5 percent (row 10).

The other columns use alternate scenarios to illustrate further the dependence of estimated price change on the value of additional quality. In the scenario in column 3, outcome improves by only a small amount, so price rises (though by quite different percentage amounts) under all three measures. In column 4, as noted, price is unchanged if the physical measure is used but does change using the other measures. The last column describes a scenario in which there is a relatively large improvement in quality, so that price is estimated to fall under all but the lowest value ($10) measure.

The main point of this exercise is not to argue that either type of measure is perfect, or even necessarily better, but rather to show that the type of measure does matter. In effect, the physical measure shows how much the price per unit of quality added is changing in one period relative to its value in the previous period, whereas the value-based measures tell us (as they were constructed to do) how much better off consumers would have been had prices not increased.

More important, the value-based measures describe the change in price of the initial product or unit, for example, an insurance policy, whereas the physical measure shows what is happening to the price of a unit of survival. The two measures reflect the price changes of different things, different bundles. I would argue, however, that the value-based measure is better when the problem is not just changing quality but changing technology. The physical measure works best when it was and is possible to buy different amounts of quality at a given "price" per unit of quality; the value-based measures work best when the improved quality is entirely new and could not have been purchased in the previous period. For instance, if automobiles increase in horsepower, we could calculate the increment in cost per horsepower added in the previous period and compare that with the cost per horsepower added in the current period. Since consumers probably could have added yet more horsepower in the previous period at the previous period's cost, we might assume that the marginal value of a unit of horsepower equaled the previous period's cost per unit added. If the cost or price per horsepower added rose, we would say that prices increased. However, most technical change in medical care provides options that are entirely new. Then, as in the case of Baumgardner's serious illness, it is quite possible for new medical technology to be worth much more than its cost, even if the cost per physical measure is rising.

This issue is related to a paradox in cost-effectiveness analysis: when two interventions are mutually exclusive, the one with the lower cost-effectiveness ratio is not necessarily preferred. For instance, if program A provides one additional QALY at a cost of $1, and program B provides 100 QALYs at a cost of $1,000, program B may still be preferred— if the *value* of the additional ninety-nine QALYS is greater than the additional cost of $999. Obviously, this assumes that one cannot produce the additional QALYs by repeating program A ninety-nine more times. In the same way, adding a new technology to an insurance package may lower the (willingness-to-pay) quality-adjusted premium even if the cost per QALY in the addition is higher than the previous values of cost per QALY, as long as the value per QALY is greater than the cost *and* there is no way other than the new technology to obtain the additional QALYs.

What to Do and How to Do It Well

This chapter is intended to be conceptual, not applied, so I will not go into great detail on the question of advantages and disadvantages of competing alternative measures. As already noted, the measurement tasks (like most worthwhile tasks) will be difficult. I believe the greatest difficulty will be describing and evaluating the change in a technology that has a variety of effects.

As I have already indicated, the most frequently used measure of changing technology in medical care is a residual: what is left of increasing expenditures after changes in population, demographics, illness incidence, and the (old) price index are taken into account. Even nonexperts know that there have been some major changes in medical technology, usually embodied in a costly and prominent piece of capital equipment (magnetic resonance imaging), new drugs (cholesterol-lowering drugs), or new medical techniques (stents). Although obviously somewhat imprecise, attempts to relate such clear changes to the residual measure usually conclude that only a minority of the residual can be attributed to these identified technologies. We suspect that the remaining part represents diffusion of old technologies and "social services" technologies, such as discharge planning.

Generally speaking, any measure of quality change due to technology might perform two tasks: *combination* and *valuation*. The combination task is unavoidable. If a change in technology affects both survival and some other characteristic consumers value, or just multiple quality-of-life characteristics, some method must be used to combine these disparate physical measures into a single measure of effectiveness. Contingent valuation techniques, in theory, perform this task effortlessly and directly: people simply report what they will pay for the new product, with all of its characteristics.

When one uses physical effectiveness measures, such as QALYs, the task is more complex. One much debated issue in determining how to obtain valid weights to convert survival into quality of life is whom to ask. Should a set of patients with the condition in question be asked about their hypothetical trade-offs, or should a random sample of the population express the trade-offs they would make if they had the condition? In part differences may arise because of different degrees of familiarity with the disease and treatment options, but it may also be that, because of attitudes toward risk and differences in current "endowments" of survival probability, trade-offs may differ even among equally well informed people. Researchers do make a choice of subjects but usually not with any particular persuasive rationale.

Willingness-to-pay measures avoid some of this arbitrariness. If the measure to be used is the willingness to pay an insurance premium, people who are or might be in the market for health insurance are the right ones to ask. There may still be some problems if the change in health is large, or if many people who might experience the benefit are not currently in the market; either way, their values may not be marginal values.

A second problem with QALY measures concerns the validity and reliability of the reported trade-off between quantity and quality of life. These trade-offs may be measured in a number of different ways—using an analog scale, a set of standard gambles, or a hypothetical time trade-off. The problem is that research shows that these three techniques usually give quite different answers—so which answer is correct? Some analysts prefer the standard gamble weights because of the consistency of this method with the economist's version of expected utility theory, but it may not be valid to assume that consumers all are or should be little economic theorists. Again a choice, somewhat arbitrary, must be made. In theory, the trade-off someone would be willing to make between the quantity of life (survival) and the quality of life (avoiding morbidity) should equal the ratio of the willingness to pay for survival to the willingness to pay to remedy quality-of-life reductions—so there is nothing special about the QALYs method for weighting unlikes. (One could just as well have measured the quality of an automobile in terms of expected miles of survival [until junking], and treated air conditioning and cup holders in terms of the lifetime expected miles buyers would be willing to sacrifice in order to get them.) Finally, the assumptions on the form of the utility function needed to make the QALYs approach appropriate are actually quite restrictive and, in any event, the willingness to trade off quantity of life for quality of life appears to vary (directly) with the level of life expectancy.

A third matter goes more directly to the question of the validity of measurement. There are some preventable medical events that involve short periods of intense pain or discomfort. However, generally such periods receive minimal weights in terms of lifetime discounted quality-adjusted life-years, if they only last for a day or a week. In contrast, people may well be willing to pay sizable amounts to avoid brief but intense pain. Economists would urge that such preferences should be manifested in the quality-of-life measure, but in reality they are not, because such survival-based measures are very insensitive to anything that affects well-being for only a small fraction of the total period of survival.

Finally, the QALYs approach does not completely adjust the physical measure for either the riskiness of the outcome or the preferences of the consumer toward risk. There is no doubt that people attach different values to a given number of expected life-years, depending on the risk characteristics of the situation. Especially when QALYs are aggregated, however, this detail is lost. There is an alternative measure that is used—defining the outcome of any intervention in terms of its (certain) healthy year equivalent, but this measure is not common.[16]

All of these problems arise not because developers of the QALY approach were obtuse or neglectful but because that approach places a premium on the task of aggregating unlikes into a single measure, for practical reasons of data collection, feasibility, economy, and comparability. For the original purpose of these measures—program evaluation with a fixed budget—these properties are not necessarily harmful, in part because there are relatively few close calls. (The measures of statistical significance or estimation precision appropriate to use in such circum-

16. See Mehrez and Gafni (1990) on the alternative measure.

stances is an issue, of course.) However, for purposes of constructing a reliable price index, these usually inconsequential flaws become much more prominent.

The most common objection to willingness-to-pay measures, that they are biased in favor of higher-income persons, usually does not apply to the case of price indexes. Most obviously, various versions of the CPI are constructed based on the market basket and well-being of people in specified circumstances. For instance, CPI-W is intended to apply only to urban workers. This family's evaluation of quality may be greater than that of low-income unemployed persons, and lower than that of a high-income entrepreneur, but those persons are not included in this measure.

Even if we do make comparisons or calculate averages across populations that vary by income class, how serious any dependence of willingness to pay on income will be will depend on the use anticipated for the quality-adjusted CPI index. Suppose it is used (as is common) to adjust transfer payments for low-income persons upward and taxes for higher-income persons downward. If higher valuation for quality by the well-to-do does occur, the use of a willingness-to-pay measure, based on value for each income class, will tend to lead to higher estimated rates of price growth for low-income people and lower rates of price growth for higher-income people. Compared to an approach that used QALYs of uniform monetary value, transfer payments will be increased for the poor and taxes would be higher for the rich. Using willingness to pay to value quality generally will not lead to inequitable effects of the CPI; if anything, the result will be more favorable to the poor than using a QALY measure, which will understate the adverse effect of inflation on poor people.

How Much Change and How Much Rationality?

The message so far is that it appears possible to produce credible willingness-to-pay–based estimates of the value of medical services quality improvements, especially when those improvements per time period are relatively small and well specified. Little has been done to value quality that substantially affects health for a specific subpopulation, or for the entire vector of quality changes, across all diseases, that occurs in reality.

Perhaps a valuable plan for research would produce valid valuation techniques for privately consumed medical care that could be used both for (specific) program evaluation and for computing price and real consumption measures. How would such a measure be derived, and how could we tell whether it was valid? My suggestion is that the *object* of valuation be defined as the difference between the willingness to pay premiums for a managed care plan covering all of the technology available in the preceding period and the willingness to pay for the same plan covering the technology available in the current period.

The consumer's evaluation problem is both complex and, in a world of voluntary insurance, unavoidable. It is complex because the consumer must know or estimate both the probabilities of needing to use the new technology and the benefit from that technology. But since refusing to adopt the new technology is a strategy available to any plan, a consumer choosing among plans will have to be able to make this evaluation in any case, well or poorly. Thus in contrast to evaluation of public goods like environmental quality changes, health insurance consumers should in principle be familiar with (if not happy with) the actual trade-off or choice being proposed.

In any year, the technologies to heal many diseases change. The change in technology represented by insurance plan coverage then represents a mix of changes for illness or conditions with different probabilities, some potentially interacting. Might it not be better, one might ask, to follow a disease- or condition-specified approach, asking about valuations one at a time?

The primary advantage to such an approach is clarity and simplicity. Both the determination of what really did change in the technical process and the valuation of that change could be kept specific and focused, avoiding the danger of contamination by other subjects or by general sentiments about whether new technology is valuable. However, research on contingent valuation in health care and in other areas suggests two problems. The most general one is a kind of "adding up" problem: people often report willingness to pay for a bundle of changes that is not much greater than what they report for individual components of the bundle. Sometimes this phenomenon, especially in the environmental area, reflects what is called the "embedding problem": people may be using their responses to questions about specific programs to express their general attitudes toward the policy in question: environmental protection, in one case, or improved medical technology, in another. In this sense, their response to a question about the value of insurance coverage of a specific new technology may reflect (if it reflects anything at all) their value of new technology in general, or just the sentiment that they would be willing to pay something more to get it. "Batching" avoids the embedding problem by requiring the respondent to consider the relevant *set* of new technologies. There should be much less of an adding-up problem when the respondent is forced to confront the total change in the premium.

The other advantage of the managed care premium approach is that it directly incorporates attitudes toward risk. Imagine that there are two new technologies that improve the expected value of health to the same extent, but one does so for a condition that is virtually certain to happen (for example, the common cold) and the other does so for a condition that is rare and catastrophic (so that the absolute increase in health, conditional on the occurrence of illness, is larger in the second case). I believe it is likely that the value of the second technology will be greater than that of the first if people are, in some general sense, risk averse. Because of risk aversion, people insure medical care costs, especially for the second type of illness. Indeed, if the cost of the treatment for the second type of illness is large relative to the person's income, willingness to pay at the point of use might be much more affected by lower income than would willingness to pay additional managed care premiums.

My conclusion then is that the "marginal premium value" applied to the set or the batch of new technologies managed care plans supply is the best measure, from the set of possible cost-effectiveness and cost-benefit measures, to use for the purpose of constructing a more accurate general medical price index.

A Hedonic Measure?

Might it be possible to measure the value of quality by comparing the actual market premiums associated with different levels of technology? Probably not, at least not until we get some more experience with this approach. As noted above, *if* one thought that insurance buyers were purchasing in a well-functioning market, then this type of data would be useful. One would still need to identify a plan offering "last year's technology at this year's prices," to get an estimate of the pure price change.

There are, however, two potential impediments to using such market data, both dealing with the employment-related group, which is the setting for the great bulk of American insurance purchases. First, these purchases are subject to a tax subsidy, so the valuation would reflect this tax loophole. In addition, there is the question of whether the corporate buyer is well informed and well motivated—especially whether the firm takes account of the diversity of preferences of its employees.[17] Because it distorts markets, the tax subsidy to employment-related health insurance makes even price index measurement more difficult than it should be.

Conclusion

Analysts face trade-offs in devising quality measures for medical interventions with which to generate improved measures of pure price change. In effect, the choice is between a contingent valuation–based measure that will try to measure precisely the right thing in a way known to be imprecise and a physical outcome measure that will probably generate a more precise measure of something only imprecisely correlated with (or correlatable with) the correct measure. Again, as is often the case, which measure one should choose on theoretical grounds depends on one's objectives. For analysis of expenditure changes for populations heavily subsidized by public programs—Medicaid and the part of Medicare spending that goes to low-income elderly—it may be best to use the monetized QALYs approach, precisely because the monetization, as well as the entire program, is really an object of collective choice. There is little point, say, in adjusting Medicaid spending for the value Medicaid beneficiaries place on improved quality, even if we knew it. Since the rationale for these programs is primarily altruistic externalities, we might as well let the altruists value the quality change.

Public programs for poor people probably account for little more than one-tenth of all national health care expenditures. What of the rest? If one is interested in constructing measures of pure price change for individual diseases or treatments that have potentially been subject to technical change, the use of physical measures, then monetized, may be appropriate *if* the physical measure itself is appropriate. For instance, if it is known that the only effect of technical change is to change survival from some disease or treatment, using a physical measure is more sensible than in the alternative case in which outcomes affected are multidimensional, not limited to health, and subject to risk variation. Moreover, if a precise measure of pure price change is not desired, but rather only a test of the hypothesis that such change is above or below some level (such as zero), using expert or subjective but reasonable approximations to the value of survival may be good enough.

17. Pauly (1997).

Conversely, where one desires a numerically precise measure in a situation with multiple and multidimensional technical changes, the contingent evaluation approach, for all its procedural tentativeness, may be the most advisable. One kind of research that would be helpful here would be an investigation of whether, in practice, the two approaches would yield substantially divergent results. Perhaps they would not if, by chance, when averaged across the kind of technical change we actually have had (and will have), a QALY-type measure is reasonably accurate (errors cancel out), and the expert judgment, labor market–based, or subjective choice of values actually match the monetary values consumers would place on them. That is, if we can determine that the monetized physical measures approaches are indeed a reasonable approximation of the value of quality improvement, they would (at present, in any case) be easier and less controversial to implement than contingent valuation measures. Of course, the suggested comparative study could only convey bad news for policy—if the correlation was not high. But at least then we would know what we do not know about medical services price changes and why we do not know it.

References

Appel, Lawrence J., and others. 1990. "Risk Reduction from Low Osmolality Contrast Media: What Do Patients Think It Is Worth?" *Medical Care* 28(4): 324–37.

Baumgardner, James. 1991. "The Interaction between Forms of Insurance Contract and Types of Technical Change in Medical Care." *Rand Journal of Economics* 22: 36–53.

Berndt, Ernst R., Iain M. Cockburn, and Zvi Griliches. 1996. "Pharmaceutical Innovations and Market Dynamics: Tracking Effects on Price Indexes for Antidepressant Drugs." *Brookings Papers on Economic Activity.* Microeconomics Supplement (*Microeconomics*): 133–99.

Cummings, Ronald G., David S. Brookshire, and William D. Schulze. 1986. *Valuing Environmental Goods: An Assessment of the Contingent Valuation Method.* Totowa, N.J.: Rowman and Allanheld.

Diamond, Peter A., and Jerry A. Hausman. 1994. "Contingent Valuation: Is Some Number Better than No Number?" *Journal of Economic Perspectives* 8(4): 45–64.

Donaldson, Cam, and Phil Shackley. 1997. "Does 'Process Utility' Exist? A Case Study of Willingness to Pay for Laparoscopic Cholecystectomy." *Social Science and Medicine* 44(5): 699–707.

Eastaugh, Steven R. 1991. "Valuation of the Benefits of Risk-Free Blood: Willingness to Pay for Hemoglobin Solutions." *International Journal of Technology Assessment in Health Care* 7(1): 51–57.

Fuchs, Victor R. 1996. "Economics, Values, and Health Care Reform." *American Economic Review* 86: 1–24.

Gafni, Amiram. 1991. "Willingness to Pay as a Measure of Benefits: Relevant Questions in the Context of Public Decisionmaking about Health Care Programs." *Medical Care* 29(12): 1246–52.

Goddeeris, John H. 1984. "Medical Insurance, Technological Change, and Welfare." *Economic Inquiry* 22(1): 56–67.

Gold, Marthe R., and others. 1996. *Cost-Effectiveness in Health and Medicine.* New York: Oxford University Press.

Johannesson, Magnus. 1992. "Economic Evaluation of Lipid Lowering: A Feasibility Test of the Contingent Valuation Approach." *Health Policy* 20: 309–20.

Johannesson, Magnus, Bengt Johnsson, and Lars Borquist. 1991. "Willingness to Pay for Antihypertensive Therapy: Results of a Swedish Pilot Study." *Journal of Health Economics* 10: 461–73.

Johannesson, Magnus, and Milton C. Weinstein. 1993. "On the Decision Rules of Cost-Effectiveness Analysis." *Journal of Health Economics* 12: 459–67.

Kartman, Bernt, Fredrik Andersson, and Magnus Johannesson. 1996. "Willingness to Pay for Reductions in Angina Pectoris Attacks." *Medical Decision Making* 16(3): 248–53.

Levit, Katherine R., and others. 1996. "National Health Expenditures, 1994." *Health Care Financing Review* 17(3): 205–42.

Lindholm, Lars, Måns Rosen, and Gideon Hellsten. 1994. "Are People Willing to Pay for a Community-Based Preventive Program?" *International Journal of Technology Assessment* 10(2): 317–24.

Mehrez, Abraham, and Amiram Gafni. 1990. "Evaluating Health Related Quality of Life: An Indifference Curve Interpretation for the Time Trade-off Technique." *Social Science and Medicine* 31: 1281–83.

Meltzer, David. 1997. "Accounting for Future Costs in Medical Cost-Effectiveness Analysis." *Journal of Health Economics* 16(1): 33–64.

O'Brien, Bernie J., and others. 1998. "Assessing the Value of a New Pharmaceutical: A Feasibility Study of Contingent Valuation in Managed Care." *Medical Care* (in press).

Pauly, Mark V. 1997. *Health Benefits at Work: An Economic and Political Analysis of Employment-Related Health Insurance.* University of Michigan Press.

Phelps, Charles E., and Alvin I. Mushlin. 1991. "On the (Near) Equivalence of Cost-Effectiveness and Cost-Benefit Analyses." *International Journal of Technology Assessment in Health Care* 7(1): 12–21.

Ramsey, Scott D., and others. 1997. "Willingness to Pay for Antihypertensive Care: Evidence from a Staff-Model HMO." *Social Science and Medicine* 44(12): 1911–17.

Reder, Melvin. 1969. "Some Problems in the Measurement of Productivity in the Medical Care Industry." In *Production and Productivity in the Service Industries,* edited by Victor Fuchs. Columbia University Press for the National Bureau of Economic Research (NBER).

Ryan, Mandy, Julie Ratcliffe, and Janet Tucker. 1997. "Using Willingness to Pay to Value Alternative Models of Antenatal Care." *Social Science and Medicine* 44(3): 371–80.

Sugden, Richard, and Alan Williams. 1978. *The Principles of Practical Cost-Benefit Analysis.* Oxford University Press.

Viscusi, W. Kip. 1993. "The Value of Risks to Life and Health." *Journal of Economic Literature* 31: 1912–46.

Zelthraseus, Niklas, and others. 1997. "The Impact of Hormone Replacement Therapy on Quality of Life and Willingness to Pay." *British Journal of Obstetrics and Gynecology* 104: 1191–95.

7

Accounting for Health Care: Integrating Price Index and Cost-Effectiveness Research

Jack E. Triplett

PERSONAL HEALTH CARE expenditures in the National Health Accounts increased at an average annual rate of 10.2 percent per year between 1985 and 1992. Whether or not health care prices were also rising rapidly between 1985 and 1992 is less clear.

Health expenditures are the product of price and quantity. Determining whether expenditure increases are caused by price increases requires a methodology for separating health care spending into price and quantity changes—into medical price inflation and increases in the output of health care. Economic statisticians lack an adequate methodology for this task.

For the same reason, it is also not clear why the United States commits 14 percent of gross domestic product to health care, a far larger share than any other major industrialized country. Does the U.S. health care sector have inefficiently high costs, as some seem to believe? Or in significant ways does the United States provide a higher level of health care than other countries with which it is compared? Better methodology for separating health care spending into price and quantity components would provide information to answer these questions.

Inadequate economic measurement can have serious consequences for health care policy analysis and for public debate. When economic statistics for the health care sector do not accurately separate price from quantity, health policy actions undertaken to suppress presumed medical price inflation will be inappropriate if the quantities are rising and the output of medical care is expanding. Separating price from quantity is not the end of the story: It has also been asserted that the United States

220

employs too many complicated medical procedures (that is, the quantities are too many). But partitioning medical expenditure into price and output change is clearly necessary for subsequent analysis.

Background

Accounting for price and quantity change in health care is an old problem that has been discussed repeatedly in the price index literature and in medical economics. Historically, the medical care price index of the CPI has been used to measure medical inflation. This index's methodology has also determined the concepts for measuring medical care output, because output measures are typically produced through deflation—that is, by dividing the change in expenditures by a price index. In the United States, medical care output measures appear in the National Income and Product Accounts (NIPA), published by the Bureau of Economic Analysis, and the National Health Accounts (NHA), published by the Health Care Financing Administration.

The CPI medical care index was until recently constructed from a sample of medical care transactions: a hospital room rate, the price for administering a frequently prescribed medicine, or the charge for a visit to a doctor's office. Transactions of this kind are sufficiently standardized that the same transaction can be observed repeatedly, which is required for a monthly price index.

It was widely noted, even thirty-five years ago, that CPI methodology did not adequately allow for improvements in medical care. For several reasons, an improvement in medical procedures that raised the cost of treatment but also improved efficacy frequently showed up as an increase in the CPI medical care component. When this CPI component was used as a deflator, the improved medical care procedure was thereby inappropriately removed from the medical output measure.

An early alternative to CPI methodology was the idea of pricing the "cost of a cure," estimating the cost of a medical procedure (the treatment of appendicitis, for example). George Stigler, in testimony on the Stigler Committee Report, remarked that "we were impressed by some of the preliminary work that has been done . . . on problems such as the changing cost of the treatment of a specific medical ailment. . . .We think it would be possible . . . to take account of things such as the much more rapid recovery and the much shorter hospital stay."[1] This contrasted with

---

1. U.S. Congress (1961), p. 533.

the CPI's focus on hospital billing elements for a medical procedure, such as the hospital room rate and the administration of a pain medication.

Scitovsky, using data collected from hospitals, estimated the cost of treating selected medical conditions, including appendicitis and otitis media, and compared the cost trends with the CPI. Her findings, though, did not confirm CPI upward bias, a result that most economists regarded as puzzling.[2] Rice and Horowitz reported on a special study conducted by the Bureau of Labor Statistics (BLS); again, the study indicated that prices for a selected group of surgical and hospital procedures rose less than the CPI physicians' fee index and the CPI medical care services component.[3] The study covered only fifteen months, bridging the time that Medicare first became operational. Few similar cost-of-illness studies have been conducted until quite recently.

Reder proposed bypassing the medical care pricing problem altogether by pricing medical insurance: "If medical care is that which can be purchased by means of medical care insurance, then its 'price' varies proportionately with the price of such insurance."[4] Barzel estimated an insurance measure of medical price inflation, using Blue Cross–Blue Shield plans.[5] Feldstein objected that the cost of insurance approach "is almost certain to be biased upward" because "average premiums will rise through time in reflection of the trend toward more comprehensive coverage" and because the insurance plans will purchase "more services or services of higher quality."[6] Moreover, if an epidemic occurs that raises the cost of insurance (AIDS, for example), it will inappropriately show up as an increase in the price of medical care and, therefore, not an increase in its quantity, unless the medical premium were calculated net of utilization rates. It is now generally recognized that measuring the output of insurance is also hard conceptually, so using insurance as a proxy is not an attractive solution to the problem of measuring health care. [7] Indeed, HMOs and capitation plans pose more difficult measurement problems than traditional fee-for-service provision of health care.

2. Scitovsky (1967) suggested that the CPI had understated the rate of medical inflation because actual average charges had advanced relative to the "customary" charges that presumably went into the CPI. In recent years, it has been asserted that the error from "list" prices goes the other way—it raises the CPI relative to the true rate of medical inflation; see Newhouse (1989).

3. Rice and Horowitz (1967).

4. Reder (1969), p. 98.

5. Barzel (1969).

6. Feldstein (1969), p. 141.

7. Griliches (1992).

As these references from the 1960s suggest, the major issues on health care output have long been joined. Until recently, the debate on the measurement of prices and output in the medical sector largely repeated the arguments of thirty years ago. The empirical work and the data, too, had not gone that much beyond the mid-1960s.[8]

Recently there have been several changes. First, in 1992 in the producer price index and in 1997 in the CPI, the Bureau of Labor Statistics introduced new medical price indexes that are substantial improvements on what existed before.[9] But the basic problem remains. If, for example, a better but more expensive treatment for heart attacks becomes available, the more costly treatment will probably show up as medical price inflation unless the BLS can get hospitals to place a value on the improved treatment, which hospitals typically cannot do.

Second, a major new research initiative on health care price indexes, using new approaches and new sources of data, has been undertaken by a research group centered in the National Bureau of Economic Research. Examples are chapters 2 and 3 of this volume.

Third, information on health care outcomes has been enhanced greatly by recent research on cost-effectiveness analysis within the medical establishment itself. Gold and others provide a comprehensive review of cost-effectiveness procedures.[10]

The present chapter is part of a larger project directed to the task of building these new price indexes and health outcome measures into a "health account" for the medical care sector. Present accounting systems for health care are organized around an institutional framework (hospitals, doctors' offices, and so forth). In an earlier paper, I contend that improvements in measuring the price and output of medical care can best be made by shifting away from this institutional orientation toward cost-of-disease accounting, of the type pioneered in the United States by Rice and recently expanded and updated by Hodgson and Cohen, and by constructing cost-of-disease accounts in a time series context, as are other accounting systems (time series comparability has not been a priority for cost-of-disease accounts in the past).[11] Cost-of-disease accounts can make use of economic information for specific diseases, such as price indexes for heart attacks (see chapter 2) and mental depression (see chapter 3), for example, and of information on cost effectiveness of

8. Newhouse (1989).
9. Cardenas (1996); Catron and Murphy (1996).
10. Gold and others (1996).
11. Hodgson and Cohen (1998); Rice (1966); and Triplett (1998).

alternative treatments for specific diseases. It is much harder to use this information in an accounting system for, say, expenditures in doctors' offices.

Studies on price indexes for diseases and cost-effectiveness studies on treatments for diseases have so far been conducted independently, with no interaction between them. Combining information from those two sources of information requires an analytic framework for how they fit together. Filling this gap is the subject of this chapter.

Comparing Price Index and Cost-Effectiveness Methods

A matrix of hypothetical health care information is given in table 7-1. I will use this information to demonstrate the relation between price indexes and cost-effectiveness research.

The subject of table 7-1 is a particular disease, a code or classification from the International Classification of Diseases, 9th revision, or ICD-9.[12] An example of an ICD classification is ICD-9 code 410, acute myocardial infarction, or heart attack, which has been the subject of considerable research, encompassing both price index research and cost-effectiveness studies.[13] ICD-9 code 410 is located in chapter 7 of ICD-9, "Circulatory Diseases." Note that U.S. diagnostic related groups, or DRGs, can be mapped into ICD-9 codes.[14]

The rows of table 7-1 designate four alternative medical interventions for the specified disease. Two of them (treatment A and treatment B) are available in period 1; a new intervention (treatment C) becomes available in period 2, and another new one (treatment D) in period 3, at which time the oldest and (by specification, for purposes of the example) least effective treatment (treatment A) is no longer employed.

In the cells of table 7-1, four types of information are recorded. The first piece of information is the transaction price for each treatment in each period—p_{a1} is the transaction price of treatment A in period 1, p_{a2} the price for the same treatment in period 2, and so forth. By transaction price, I mean the charge made by a medical provider for administering the specified medical intervention. The medical price index literature is full of discussions about the difficulty of obtaining the transactions price (as opposed to the list or "chargemaster" price) and about whether "the"

12. Puckett (1997).
13. See chapter 2 of this volume on price index research.
14. *Diagnosis Related Groups Definitions Manual* (1997).

Table 7-1. *Matrix of Hypothetical Health Care*

Treatments	Period 1	Period 2	Period 3
Treatment A	$p_{a1}q_{a1}M_aV_1$	$p_{a2}q_{a2}M_aV_2$	...
Treatment B	$p_{b1}q_{b1}M_bV_1$	$p_{b2}q_{b2}M_bV_2$	$p_{b3}q_{b3}M_bV_3$
Treatment C	...	$p_{c2}q_{c2}M_cV_2$	$p_{c3}q_{c3}M_cV_3$
Treatment D	...	...	$p_{d3}q_{d3}M_dV_3$

price makes any sense, given the tendency to price discriminate among patients according to income or ability to pay or class of payer. It is also the case that much variation exists among the medical conditions of patients who may fall into the same ICD-9, or DRG, code, and this variation affects the treatment, its cost, and therefore the amount charged. I abstract from these considerations, without implying in any way that I denigrate their importance and relevance or the intractability of the problems they present. If necessary, one can think of the p terms in the table as "average transactions prices."

The treatment methods are arrayed in table 7-1 from the least expensive to the most expensive, that is, $p_{at} < p_{bt} < p_{ct} < p_{dt}$, for each time period, t. This implies that new methods are always more expensive than old ones and also that when treatment methods go out of use, they are the less expensive ones (compare the arrays for periods 2 and 3).[15] It is not necessary to make any assumption about the movement over time of prices for a given treatment, but the exposition will be easier, and probably more realistic, if we assume that prices for each treatment, i, are increasing over time, that is $p_{i1} < p_{i2} < p_{i3}$.

The second piece of information in each cell of table 7-1 is the quantity of each medical procedure that is performed in each time period. Thus, q_{b2} is the number of treatment B procedures performed in period 2, and so forth. The pattern of table 7-1 suggests that newer treatments enter with small shares and expand and that older ones have declining shares and are eventually supplanted. This is consistent with the shares of treatment regimens shown in Cutler and others.[16] However, the patterns of relative quantities and their changes are not crucial for present purposes.

The third and fourth pieces of information are a medical outcome measure (M_i), which is unique to a specific treatment but does not depend

15. Frank, Berndt, and Busch (chapter 3 of this volume) present a counter-example, a new and equally effective treatment that is far cheaper than the old one.
16. Chapter 2.

on time, and a valuation of the medical outcome (V_t), which does vary with time but, ideally, is not unique to the treatment (provided the M_i terms are measured correctly). These will be described and considered when I make use of them, at a later point.

Conventional Price Indexes and Output Measures

By "conventional price index," I mean price indexes of the type now produced by the Bureau of Labor Statistics, in which the pricing unit is, in effect, a specified treatment for a defined medical condition. I noted earlier that the CPI medical care price index was once (before January 1997) formed from the price of a hospital room, and so forth, and that the BLS recently has moved to an improved approach. In the current CPI (and in the producer price index, the PPI), the BLS first takes a sample of medical procedures (actually, of DRGs). It then samples, from among all the cases in a hospital or physician's office records, an individual patient's bill (or bills). The characteristics of the patient and of the treatment are specified in great detail. The agency then collects the charges in subsequent periods for the precisely specified medical case that was chosen in the initial period.[17]

A statistical agency is not likely to produce a price index at so disaggregate a level as an ICD-9 three-digit code, so the following should not be taken as an explicit description of any country's methodology for health price indexes. The BLS, however, does produce PPI indexes at the level of an ICD-9 chapter (for example, "Circulatory Diseases"). The principles can be illustrated efficiently by assuming a price index for a more narrowly specified category (ICD-9 code 410—heart attack).

Suppose, then, that the statistical agency has decided to construct a price index covering all the treatments in table 7-1. Typically, the agency will choose a sample. Although sampling has substantial importance in practice, sampling considerations are not particularly relevant to the present discussion. The array of data in table 7-1 will illustrate the basic problems of constructing price indexes, whether done with samples of treatments or with an exhaustive survey of them.

Statistical agencies typically use the Laspeyres formula to compute the price change for medical treatments. A Laspeyres price index weights the

---

17. See Catron and Murphy (1996). This BLS procedure is not necessarily employed by the statistical offices of other countries. Very few countries, for example, do probability sampling of price quotations for price indexes.

change in each of the prices by the number employed of each treatment in period 1.[18] Symbolically, the calculating formula for this price index (which I denote with a capital letter, P) is:

$$(7\text{-}1) \qquad P_{12} = \Sigma p_{i2}\, q_{i1}/\Sigma p_{i1}\, q_{i1}.$$

Note that the price measure holds constant the treatment (and other aspects of the hospital or physician encounter), so the comparisons that are made for the price index are exclusively across the rows of table 7-1.

In the Laspeyres calculation, only period 1 quantities, q_{i1}, are employed. In period 1, two treatments only are available, A and B. The new treatment, C, was not available in period 1, so no use is made of the period 2 quantities, q_{i2}. Accordingly, treatment C can have no role in the price index calculation of equation (7-1)—it has no price index weight in period 1 because $q_{c1} = 0$. This is not an innocuous point but rather a potentially serious source of error to which I will return.

The next step is constructing an output measure for medical treatments. It is generally true that output measures in economic statistics are calculated indirectly. Output, or quantity, measures are estimated through deflation by a price index. The principles are as follows.

National accountants, and particularly national health accountants, go to great lengths to collect, estimate, and record total national expenditure on medical treatments.[19] In our example, this is simply the aggregate spending in period 1 on the two treatments that were available in period 1; similarly, total expenditure in period 2 is the aggregate spending on the three treatments that were available in period 2. Algebraically, these two expenditures amount to (using the information in table 7-1):

$$(7\text{-}2a) \qquad \text{Exp}_1 = \Sigma p_{i1}\, q_{i1}, i = a,b$$

$$(7\text{-}2b) \qquad \text{Exp}_2 = \Sigma p_{i2}\, q_{i2}, i = a,b,c.$$

18. Actually, at this level the agency typically does not have expenditure weights, though it may have sampling weights, the use of which will give the same formula, as an expectation. It might also use alternative calculations, including a geometric mean, rather than the arithmetic mean implied by equation 7-1. The best method for calculating such "basic components" in price indexes is a topic that is currently the subject of substantial professional debate; the subject cannot be pursued here.

19. Lazenby and others (1992).

The ratio of (7-2b) to (7-2a) gives the change in expenditure between the two periods, which in national accounts language (at least in the United States) is often called the change in "current dollar" expenditure.[20]

In national accounts, the change in current dollar expenditure is "deflated" by the appropriate price index to obtain the change in output, which is a quantity change measure. I will denote this quantity change measure with a capital letter, Q. Then, the change in output between periods 1 and 2 is: [21]

$$(7\text{-}3) \qquad\qquad Q_{12} = (\text{Exp}_2 / \text{Exp}_1) / P_{12}.$$

An important property of this conventional deflation method is: the change in the output of medical procedures between periods 1 and 2 *includes* the output of treatment C in period 2, even though, as noted above, the price index that is used for deflation *does not include* treatment C. Including treatment C in the output measure makes sense because the quantity of treatment C went from zero in period 1 to some positive number of treatments, designated by q_{c2}, in period 2. However, the introduction of the "higher quality" treatment C is outside the CPI sample, it is not included in the CPI. Thus, treatment C's quantity increase in national accounts is implicitly valued by the prices for treatments A and B.

It is very appropriate to ask whether the price movement for treatments A and B provides a valid basis for valuing the quantity increase in treatment C. The greater an improvement treatment C is over treatments A and B, the more dubious the use of prices for treatments A and B to value the increase in the quantity of treatment C.

---

20. In the usual presentation, the ratio is converted to a percentage increase or decrease by subtracting 1 from the ratio, or: (Exp2 / Exp1) − 1 = percent change in expenditures.

21. Readers who are well versed in national accounts practices will note that the algebra in equation 7-3 results in an unfamiliar expression. Statistical agencies that produce price statistics will almost always use index weights from the earlier period, as shown in equation 7-1, and will also typically hold the weights fixed over a number of periods (often called a "base-period weighted" index). When the base-period weighted (or Laspeyres) price index is used as a deflator, as in this example, the result is a current-period weighted quantity index, usually called a "Paasche" index (this is apparent from substituting equations 7-1 and 7-2 into equation 7-3). This differs from the traditional "upper-level" aggregation structure of national accounts for most countries of the world, where the upper level corresponds to a Laspeyres quantity index and a Paasche implicit deflator. It also differs from the approach introduced by the Bureau of Economic Analysis in 1996, in which both the quantity measure and the price measure are described by a different index number formula, the Fisher Ideal index number (*Survey of Current Business*, January–February 1996). But at the very lowest level of national accounts, the implicit weighting structure for output measures is determined by the formula for the deflating indexes, which is what is represented in equation 7-3.

In the price index literature, this problem is known, somewhat inappropriately, as the "new good" problem. [22] With conventional price index procedures and conventional national accounts procedures, there is a real danger that the introduction of new goods will be undervalued when the price movements of existing goods are used for valuing the new ones. A discussion of the economic measurement problems posed by new goods is contained in the "introduction" to Bresnahan and Gordon's *Economics of New Goods.*[23]

In period 3, another price index problem arises that I will describe briefly to avoid confusion by its omission. A new treatment (treatment D) becomes available in period 3, and an old treatment (A) is no longer used, so it disappears from the data that are collected for price indexes and national accounts.

The introduction of treatment D in period 3 is exactly parallel to the introduction of treatment C in period 2. However, presuming that the price index sample contains treatment A, the disappearance of treatment A requires that the price-compiling agency carry out an "item replacement" within the price index sample.[24] All commonly used methods for dealing with item replacements create potential errors in price indexes, some of which are discussed below.

In summary, the essence of the traditional price index method is to use only the prices of matched treatments—the method holds constant the characteristics of the medical intervention and the other terms of the transaction. Price comparisons are made only within rows of table 7-1. Any change in medical costs that arises outside a particular row is ignored.

Cost-Effectiveness Measures

Cost-effectiveness studies and price index studies have very different purposes. Although cost-effectiveness studies may have uses for eco-

---

22. By "inappropriate" I do not mean that the subject here is a service, rather than a good. Rather, it is not clear that the four treatments in table 7-1 should be thought of as "different" services; since they all address the same problem (the treatment of a specified disease), they might better be thought of as different "quality" levels of the same service or commodity, so we should be using language such as "new variety of good" or perhaps "new quality level of service." The language gets cumbersome. I therefore use "new good" without necessarily implying that it is a commodity or service that has never been seen before, only that it has not been available in a previous time in the form in which it is made available today.

23. Bresnahan and Gordon (1997).

24. Within methodological materials published by the U.S. Bureau of Labor Statistics, this is often referred to as an "item substitution." Methods for handling item replacements in price indexes are discussed in Triplett (1997); and in Moulton and Moses (1997).

nomic analysis, the cost-effectiveness technique is mainly an analytic tool for decisionmaking.[25]

Cost-effectiveness studies use information from table 7-1, but it is somewhat different information from the information that goes into conventional price indexes and national accounts output measures. A cost-effectiveness ratio is computed from two kinds of information. The numerator contains the cost of a medical procedure. If the only cost of an illness, or of a treatment, were the charges made by physicians and hospitals, then the numerator of the cost-effectiveness ratio could be calculated from the p_{it} terms in table 7-1. I explore below cases where medical provider charges are not the full cost of an illness.

The second piece of information in cost-effectiveness studies is a measure of medical outcome, often also called a health outcome. The outcome of an operation for a life-threatening condition might be the survival probability, or the expected number of years of life prolonged by the operation. If an improved operating procedure is developed, its increment to effectiveness could be measured by increased survival probability or the increase in expected number of life-years that it generates. In table 7-1, the medical outcome associated with each treatment—however measured, but measured consistently across treatments—is designated M_i. Because I have assumed, for expository convenience, that more expensive medical treatments have higher effectiveness (though not necessarily proportionately), $M_d > M_c > M_b > M_a$.

Suppose one desired to perform a cost-effectiveness analysis on treatments B and C in table 7-1 and the study were carried out at period 2, the point at which treatment C was introduced. Then, assuming that medical provider charges are the only costs, the difference in cost for the new intervention (C), compared with the older one (B), is $p_{c2} - p_{b2}$. The increment to effectiveness (the change in medical outcome from use of treatment [C], compared with the previously best treatment [B]) is $M_c - M_b$. The cost-effectiveness ratio is then:

$$(7\text{-}4) \quad (C/E)_{cb} = (p_{c2} - p_{b2}) / (M_c - M_b).$$

Obviously, with this formulation the lower the cost-effectiveness ratio the more desirable the new treatment is relative to the older one. As Gold and others remark, "interventions that have a relatively low c/e ratio are 'good buys' and would have high priority for resources."[26]

25. Gold and others (1996).
26. Ibid., p. 27.

The literature on cost effectiveness contains a great deal of discussion about the costs that belong in the numerator of the cost-effectiveness ratio and about the way one measures medical outcomes in the denominator.

COSTS. Generally, the costs included in a cost-effectiveness study are broader and more comprehensive than the p_{it} terms of table 7-1 because the full costs of a medical procedure include more than the charges for treatment made by the hospital or physician. Recovery from a stroke may involve an extended stay in a nursing home, for example, and the patient may incur other costs, such as the value of care provided by friends and family members. "A primary objective of cost-effectiveness analysis is to incorporate a consideration of resource consumption into decisions about health care."[27] Thus, there are direct resource costs, the charges for which are made by medical care providers, including any public subsidies, and indirect costs.[28] Gold and others categorize indirect costs into use of nonhealth resources (they give as an example the use of transportation to obtain treatment), use of unpaid or informal caregiver time, and use of the patient's own time in the course of treatment.[29]

There is still debate on cost-effectiveness methodology for some aspects of cost, especially certain future costs.[30] For present purposes, particular interest attaches to the methodology applied to the cost of the patients' own time in a cost-effectiveness study. If a new medical treatment economizes on patient time, some contributors to cost-effectiveness studies have argued that the saving should be treated as a reduction in the cost of care, others that it should be treated as an increment to the effectiveness of medical treatment (see below), and still others that it makes no difference how time savings are handled in the study as long as the method is applied consistently across studies. [31]

27. Ibid., p. 176.
28. Gold and others (ibid.) argue against the use of the term "indirect" costs on the grounds that it has different interpretations in different social science literatures. Although their point is well taken, it is nevertheless standard in accounting for health costs to partition costs into those that are measured or estimated from health care provider data or from health care expenditure data (direct costs of illness) and those that must be estimated from other kinds of data, such as earnings forgone (indirect costs). Usually, the latter estimates are also less direct in terms of estimating methods than are the former ones because direct costs are "what are" estimates (the amount paid to a hospital, for example), where indirect costs are "what would have been" estimates (the earnings that would have been received had the patient not become ill).
29. An extended discussion of costs appears in Gold and others (1996), especially chap. 6.
30. See, for example, the positions taken by Garber and Phelps (1997) and Meltzer (1997) and the review of this debate by Weinstein and Manning (1997).
31. Garber and Phelps (1997).

Whatever the existing debate about the elements of cost that belong in a cost-effectiveness ratio, though, the cost concept that is used in cost-effectiveness studies is broader than the cost or price concept that is measured in traditional price indexes and national accounts. Cost-effectiveness studies, at least in principle, address the full costs of illness; price indexes typically address only the fraction of the full cost that is identified with charges made by medical providers.

EFFECTIVENESS MEASURES. Turning now to medical outcomes, many measures of effectiveness have been employed. Probability of survival or expected lifetime is one straightforward quantitative measure that, if not a comprehensive measure of medical outcome, is not inappropriate for some diseases and treatments. For example, the probability of survival from a heart attack is a very relevant measure of medical outcomes for comparisons among alternative treatments for heart attacks, and it remains relevant even if lifestyle restrictions and ability to carry out normal functions ought also to be included in the medical outcome measure.

For other medical interventions, survival probabilities may be irrelevant (orthopedic treatment of an ankle injury, for example). Indeed, as the cost-effectiveness panel remarked: "In industrialized nations, where length of life has shown steady increases over the past century, it is the improvement in quality of life produced by health care inputs that is often the truer gauge of how well the health care system is performing. For example, in evaluating the effectiveness of cholesterol screening, mortality from health disease is certainly an important outcome. But simply counting deaths, or even life-years gained, may leave out other important health outcomes, such as the morbidity repercussions of angina and heart attacks, as well as the psychological concerns that may accompany a diagnosis of hypercholesterolemia. All of these outcomes may be highly relevant in assessing the value of an intervention."[32]

As this passage suggests, a medical outcome measure should incorporate both morbidity and mortality effects into a single measure. For this purpose, the panel recommended a measure known as QALY, the "quality-adjusted life-year."[33]

For present purposes, two characteristics of QALY can be noted. First, future years of life gained are discounted in QALY. Second, QALY incorporates community preferences across various health states in order

32. Gold and others (1996), p. 84.
33. Ibid., p. 122.

to weight different changes that are brought about by medical interventions.[34]

It has been clear for many years that measures of health outcomes are a vital step in the ultimate solution to the health care measurement problem.[35] The development of the QALY and other related measures provides a solution, in principle, to some of the problems with the cost-of-illness approach that emerged in some of the early research. For example, Scitovsky discussed a new treatment for acute appendicitis that, because of potential adverse side effects, was better in some respects (or for some care recipients) but worse in others (or for other recipients).[36] Although it was not recognized at the time, the Scitovsky study showed that the outcome of a medical procedure is generally multidimensional; one cannot just consider a "cure" or the principal or primary outcome. Put another way, looking only at the cost of a unidimensional "cure" (appendicitis treatment), without considering the multidimensional attributes or characteristics of a medical procedure, could produce its own bias. Although this problem was intractable with the analytic tools available in the 1960s, it has been addressed in the medical outcome research of the past ten to fifteen years because both increased benefits of a new procedure and side effects, if any, are valued in QALY.

In practice, however, much work remains. Bailar has long cautioned that incautious application of outcome measures may distort the apparent effects of a medical treatment.[37] Their example was early detection of cancer, with survival rates after treatment as an outcome measure. Some cancers do not kill the patient; if these cancers are detected early and are treated, the treatment may appear effective in terms of patient survival, even though the untreated patient might also have had a high survival probability. This problem exists for all medical outcome measures.

SOME ADDITIONAL CONSIDERATIONS. The numerator of the cost-effectiveness ratio is time dependent. If the costs diverge for the two treatments being compared, the cost difference in the numerator of the cost-effectiveness ratio will also change. Numerators may vary across countries as well, if the structures of medical costs differ across countries.

34. For more information on the QALY measure, its limitations and research needed to improve it, see ibid., chap. 4, and the range of authors cited on p. 93. See also the DALY (disability adjusted life-year), which is approximately 1-QALY, in Murray and Lopez (1996), which also contains an extended discussion of the measurement problems.

35. See, for example, Reder (1969).

36. Scitovsky (1964, 1967).

37. Bailar and Gornick (1997).

Intertemporal changes or international differences in costs are more probable the more expansive the definition of cost. For example, the cost of family caregivers is not constant over time, certainly differs across countries, and probably does not have a constant ratio to other included costs.

For these reasons, a cost-effectiveness ratio is a calculation that is unique to one particular time and country. This causes problems because one would typically like to apply cost-effectiveness studies to at least a medium-term period and would like to apply research carried out in one country to decisions in another.

I have assumed that the denominator—the effectiveness part of a cost-effectiveness ratio—is not time dependent. That is, once a researcher has determined the difference in effectiveness between two treatments, there is no reason to assume that the difference in effectiveness will change in some future period. Likewise, if a medical procedure makes a net contribution to effectiveness in one country, one presumes that this research finding will carry over into data for another.

However, medical outcome measures do depend on medical research. New research sometimes shows that a treatment is more effective than originally estimated and sometimes less effective. This means that, even though effectiveness measures are not themselves time dependent, they are subject to revisions, sometimes large ones. Moreover, outcomes may change because a given procedure may change in its implementation or become more effective with increasing use (evidence suggests that learning by doing in operations improves the quality of outcomes). If so, a revision to the outcome measure may also be called for. Revisions are well known in national accounts but not well liked.

Garber and Phelps argue that the patient's own time may go into either the numerator or the denominator of a cost-effectiveness ratio.[38] Because the value of the patient's own time is time dependent and will not necessarily move with other changes in costs that are also time dependent, I believe it would be better to put all time-dependent costs in the same part of the cost-effectiveness ratio. This reason complements other reasons that have been advanced for putting time costs in the numerator of the ratio.[39]

I do not want to give the impression that medical outcome measures are fully developed or minimize the controversy that still exists. Many

38. Garber and Phelps (1997).
39. See Meltzer (1997).

problems limit the comprehensiveness and accuracy of medical outcome measures.[40] In part because of the problems, outcome measures have not found ready acceptance among statistical agencies that compile price indexes and construct national accounts. But there is an additional reason: statistical agency administrators are reluctant to place an economic value on life-years or on QALYs, which seems to be required.[41]

Price Indexes and Cost-Effectiveness Studies

Price indexes and cost-effectiveness studies differ in a number of ways, largely because their respective purposes differ.

A price index study is designed to produce information about larger or smaller groups of medical procedures, taken together. A price index, and its related national accounts output measure, provides information about the aggregate price and quantity movement of some set of medical treatments, probably at a level of aggregation such as an ICD-9 chapter or subchapter, although more detailed indexes are feasible. Of necessity, price index measurements abstract from the detailed movements of prices (and quantities) for individual treatments. Sometimes one also wants to measure international price and output differences prevailing at the same time; the index number procedures are similar.

A cost-effectiveness study provides information for making comparisons among treatments, not for extracting information that is common to all of them. How much better is aspirin, or angioplasty, than alternatives for treating heart attacks? Cost-effectiveness studies are not aggregative; they are designed to produce information at a detailed level—comparisons between or among alternative treatments for a disease diagnosis. For the most part, the comparisons they make are at the same time period. They are not normally designed to provide information about time trends or international differences.

Another way to compare price indexes and cost-effectiveness studies is to contrast the way they use information from table 7-1. Both types of studies make comparisons among the elements of table 7-1, but they make different comparisons.

The price index compiler always makes comparisons within the rows of table 7-1, never down the columns. A medical care price index measures changes in the prices of medical treatments over time, holding the

---

40. They are discussed in Gold and others (1996).

41. For example, Cutler, McClellan, and Newhouse, in chapter 2 of this volume, place a value on increased life expectancy in order to compute a cost-of-living index for heart attack treatments.

treatment constant. This is exactly the information within the rows. Any medical cost changes that occur because new treatments replace old ones (changes that are not within the rows of table 7-1), any price differences that arise from differences in treatments—comparisons that go down the columns of table 7-1—are excluded from the price index. They are regarded as quality change, not price change. As noted already, the within-row information that is used is exclusively the p_{it} and q_{it} data. No use is made of the M_i information in price indexes—but, of course, M_i does not vary across rows, so there is nothing useful in the across-the-row M_i.

The cost-effectiveness study, on the other hand, is intended to make comparisons *down* the columns of table 7-1. A cost-effectiveness study that compares treatments C and B, say, compares price differences and medical outcome differences between treatments, at a fixed point in time. This is exactly the information one gets by going down the columns. The cost-effectiveness ratio uses exclusively the p_i and M_i information; it normally makes no use of the q_i terms. The cost-effectiveness ratio answers a question that traditional price index methodology cannot answer: how much better, in relation to its increased cost, is treatment C relative to treatment B?

The "Quality Problem" in Medical Price Measures (and How Medical Outcome Measures Can Help to Solve It)

The biggest problem in economic accounting for medical care is how to be sure that an improvement in medical care is counted as an increase in medical output and is not counted as medical inflation. What methods can be devised to allow for improvements in medical care in price indexes and output measures? This is the medical care version of the price index "quality problem" that has long been discussed in the context of other goods and services.[42]

Four separate categories of price index "quality problem" can be distinguished. Sometimes clear distinctions have not been drawn among them in the medical economics literature.

1. *Changes in treatment methods that are not recorded by the statistical agency.* For example, a heart bypass may be employed in modern medical care of heart disease instead of medical management, which might have been the only possibility, or the predominant method, in the past; if the statistical agency fails to address the change in treatment, an error is

---

42. See, for example, Griliches (1971).

introduced into the price index and into the deflated output measure for medical care. Unnoticed change in treatment method was certainly a problem under the old CPI procedure, in which the daily charge for a hospital room was collected, because in the old CPI procedure no consideration was given to the treatment for which the patient occupied the room. This case amounts to price comparisons that shift among the rows of table 7-1 rather than price comparisons that are constructed from matched treatments (price comparisons within the rows). The new BLS procedures that track the cost of a specified medical case have undoubtedly greatly reduced or eliminated this problem.

2. *Unnoticed (by the statistical agency) improvement (or deterioration) of care, within the rows of table 7-1.* One may control for the treatment, thus avoiding the gross noncomparabilities inherent in case (1), but is a 1982 heart bypass exactly the same as a 1997 bypass? The operation has become less invasive, learning by doing has perfected the techniques (studies show that heart operations performed at hospitals by surgeons who do that operation more frequently have more satisfactory outcomes), and recovery times have diminished. How does one handle drift in the effectiveness of what may be described, in ordinary and medical language, as the "same" treatment? Notice that this is not just a price index problem. It arises in cost-effectiveness studies as well. If procedures are modified in ways that were not incorporated into the original study, the effectiveness measure will be out of date and must be redone.

Cases (1) and (2) above are the traditional ones that have been the subjects of most past discussion in the medical economics literature. Standard price index methodology restricts price comparisons to *matched* medical treatments (comparisons within the rows of table 7-1). Cases (1) and (2) both amount to errors in holding the match constant.

It has been recognized more recently in the price index literature that the restriction to within-row comparisons, although useful to prevent errors from gross noncomparabilities, may also contribute problems. When new treatments are introduced and old ones disappear, those entries and exits may imply changes in value—measured either in price or in quantity—that are not equal to what one gets from "matched" comparisons within the rows. These are cases (3) and (4):

3. *New treatments are developed and introduced.* The matched treatment method in traditional price index ignores treatment C when it first is introduced in period 2 (and treatment D in period 3). This corresponds to what might be called "quality change outside the price index sample." The matching methodology focuses attention on the match and getting

the match right and not on changes that occur outside the set of matched price quotes. To put it another way, the methodology maximizes the likelihood of collecting prices that are exact "constant quality" matches and minimizes encounters with cases of "quality change." However, ignoring C creates potential bias in the price and output measures, even though the bias may be small if (as often asserted) the quantity of the "new good" (q_{c2}) is inconsequential in the periods just after it is introduced.

4. *The exit of old treatments and their replacement in the CPI sample.* In table 7-1, treatment A exits from the price index sample in period 4. Its disappearances forces a comparison of some kind among the rows, a comparison between treatment A and some other treatment (C, say) that will replace it in the sample. This might be called "quality change inside the price index sample." A measure of relative effectiveness, or of willingness to pay—or a "quality adjustment," in usual price index terminology—is required to make this comparison.

Note that when treatment A disappears (period 3), it is not necessarily replaced in the sample by the treatment that was newly introduced in period 3 (which is treatment D); the quality problem in case (4) is logically separate from the one in case (3), because it is not necessarily a "new good" problem. But in any case, shifting the sample from A to C may be late, in the sense that the really significant change in treatments, and the really significant change in costs, might have been the introduction of treatment C some time earlier (3), well before the disappearance of treatment A forced a "quality adjustment" in the price index (4).

Both (3) and (4) require a quality adjustment. The next section discusses the use of medical outcome information to carry out adjustments in medical price indexes for improvements in medical treatments.

Using Medical Outcome Measures in Medical Care Price Indexes

When treatment A disappears and is replaced in the price index sample by treatment C (case 4), how much of its increased cost should be counted as a quality change? The entire amount (that is, $p_{c2} - p_{a2}$)? Some price index methods imply that answer, approximately, but the correct answer depends on the extent that treatment C is better than treatment A, not on the difference in their prices.

Or considering case (3), what are the implications of the introduction of treatment C for the cost of medical care? Should the index be unaffected when treatment C is introduced? The answer depends on whether the higher cost of treatment C is or is not exactly equal to the value of the quality difference between C and the previously available treatments.

Recall from above that the cost-effectiveness ratio compares the cost difference and the effectiveness difference between two treatments (equation 7-4). We express the cost differences by the p_{it} terms of table 7-1. The effectiveness differences are measures as QALYs.

Suppose that the cost-effectiveness ratio for treatment C compared with treatment A (or treatment B) equals unity. That means that treatment C's cost increase is just offset by the improvement in its effectiveness. No true price change takes place when C replaces A (case 4), or when C is added to existing treatments (case 3). The price index that measures the cost of medical care should not change in either case.

Suppose, on the other hand, that the cost-effectiveness ratio is less than unity—the cost increase when C is introduced is less than the improvement in effectiveness it brings about. This is the case that ought to prevail when a new, more effective treatment is actually adopted and comes into general use. The true cost of medical care has gone down in this case, and the price index should fall.

Now suppose the third possibility, that the cost-effectiveness ratio is greater than unity. Treatment C causes cost to rise more than effectiveness. Implementing treatment C in this circumstance is not a wise decision, but it could happen (and the frequent talk about technology-driven medical price inflation suggests a belief that it does happen). Because the cost of medical care rises when C is introduced, the price index should also rise.

A medical outcome measure, such as QALY, provides the adjustment to apply to price indexes when a new treatment is introduced or when it is encountered in compiling the price index sample.[43] One's general presumption—and good social policy—is that new treatments will be introduced when they have low cost-effectiveness ratios, when the increment they make to the cost of care is lower than the increment they make to medical effectiveness. When that favorable condition prevails, *the traditional "matched treatment" price index methodology will miss part of the medical cost reduction associated with the introduction of a new medi-*

43. A more complete discussion would cover several points: What would a consumer be willing to pay for a QALY and the fact that it depends on the income distribution? Social valuation may differ from individual valuations: the individuals wants "the best," but society may not have the resources to pay. The various concerns about willingness to pay are not unique to QALY; they apply to any quality adjustment for medical price indexes.

cal procedure; use of QALY as an adjustment will permit the price index to record the true cost decline. Conversely, if new medical techniques worsen the cost-effectiveness ratio, then matched treatment price index methodology will miss part of the increased cost of medical care; use of QALY brings this price increase into the price index.[44]

For those who are familiar with the usual price index literature on quality change, it will appear surprising that the "value" of quality change (the value of medical outcomes) did not come up. In the method for employing medical outcome information that is outlined here, I make no actual use of the V_t terms of table 7-1; I do not need to put a price on the quality-adjusted life-years. This is not parallel with what is done for nonmedical goods and services and requires further discussion.

Value of Life in Price and Output Measures

Cutler and others calculated the number of life-years extended for heart attack victims (their medical outcome measure) and then multiplied by a value of life estimate in computing their price index for heart attacks.[45]

As mentioned, there is great reluctance to put a value on lives saved or extended. Statistical agency administrators have objected to this aspect of the price index research by Cutler and others. Gold and others note that many users of cost-effectiveness studies are "uncomfortable about attaching dollar valuations to health outcomes such as life expectancy." They also note that because cost-effectiveness analysis offers much the same information as do studies that measure health outcomes, "the distinction may be more important for the sake of appearance than for its practical consequences." [46] This is essentially the point made by Phelps and Mushlin: cost-benefit analysis, which puts an explicit monetary valuation on medical outcomes, is nearly equivalent to cost-effectiveness analysis, which does not.[47]

Responding to such concerns by saying that economists routinely value human life for other purposes (regulation analysis, suits for wrongful deaths, and so forth) is no real answer. The ethical concerns are real,

44. For simplicity, I have ignored a number of complications that arise in case (3). Price index biases caused by item replacements can go either way (even when quality is improving) because the bias depends on the nature of the method used for item replacement and the paths of price change and quality improvement. See the extended discussion in Triplett (1997).

45. Chapter 2.

46. Gold and others (1996), p. 28.

47. Phelps and Mushlin (1991).

and even if we have to value lives for some purposes, the necessity for doing so does not make the choice a more comfortable one.[48]

Accordingly, there is great value to a methodology that does not require valuing human life, and the methodology of the preceding section does not. Explaining why it does not, and why "quality adjustments" for medical care are not parallel to those for nonmedical goods and services, is the topic of this section.

Suppose one were told that a new car was improved by adding an air-conditioning system that would be included in the price; one would not know how to adjust the automobile price index for the improvement unless one also knew the value of the air-conditioning system. Why does a comparable valuation requirement not hold for medical care?

One part of the answer lies in the metric for recent measures of medical outcomes, particularly QALY: outcomes always have the same units. If the medical effectiveness measure is the expected number of years of life extended, for example, the metric is always years of life. If the outcome measure is QALY, then the outcome is always measured in a QALY unit. If one improvement in the procedures for an operation increases expected years of survival and another reduces the amount of pain during recovery, both gains in medical outcome would be valued on the common QALY scale.

On the car, the quality improvement might be 10 horsepower one year, an air-conditioning system in another, and extra cupholders in the third. We have to put a value on quality changes in cars partly because air conditioners and cupholders are "apples and oranges" that can only be combined with a monetary value. There is no natural scale to determine how much "more car per car" each of these improvements implies, so economic measurement uses a "money metric" for combining dissimilar quality improvements to the car. Similarly, a computer is viewed in economic measurement as a bundle of speed and memory;[49] partly because computer speed and memory are measured in different units, changes in computer quality must be valued in money terms.

In contrast to the cases of cars and computers, the medical community has put a lot of effort into quantifying medical effectiveness, into devising a common scale that applies to different medical interventions. Years of life extended and pain relief have been put on a common scale in the QALY. Because of that common scale, economists do not have to value

48. Schelling (1968).
49. Triplett (1987).

changes in medical effectiveness in the same way—or for the same reason—that they must put a value on changes in automobile or computer quality. One can take the percentage improvement in QALY as a direct adjustment for the percentage change in cost that is associated with the change in medical technology.[50]

Another way to make the same point is to consider the V_t terms from table 7-1. I specified earlier that V does not depend on the treatment, i. Indeed, when M_i is measured on the same scale across treatments, V cannot differ across treatments. If the outcome measures M_i and M_j are both valued by V_t (multiplying both by V_t to form a quality adjustment, $M_i V_t / M_j V_t$), then V_t falls out of the ratio. It cannot affect the quality adjustment for the medical price index.

A second part of the answer lies in the nature of that increment to effectiveness that is measured by QALY. Suppose the increments to car quality were also always in the same units (one cupholder the first year, a second the next time, then a third). No economist, I suspect, would want to value the nth cupholder the same as the first, because of the familiar idea of diminishing marginal utility to increments of consumption. For this reason, in the car case one again needs to value the cupholders, indeed, to find out the value of the nth holder.

The same proposition, however, does not hold for QALY. Here the increment is always in years. Incremental years of life are attained in the future, and future incremental years are valued lower because future years need to be discounted. In measuring QALY, future years are already discounted.[51] One cannot consume additional QALYs in timeless units, as one can the services of incremental cupholders.

Many economists would argue that an extra year of life is subject to diminishing marginal utility just like everything else, that the value of the tenth year of life extended is worth less to a ninety-year-old than to a thirty-year-old person. On the same line of reasoning, living 90 percent of one's days pain free, compared to 80 percent, might be worth less than an equivalent percentage improvement for someone who is in greater discomfort. If so, one might need to value changes in QALY.

---

50. One minor reservation arises because price index quality adjustment would normally be done in ratio form, rather than in ratios of differences, as cost-effectiveness studies are usually calculated. That is, one would like the ratios pc_2/pb_2 and M_c/M_b, and not the expressions of equation 7-4. I presume that when a cost-effectiveness study is published, the basic information in it could be used to reconstruct the ratios, or that, alternatively, these calculating differences would make only a small effect on the actual calculation of the price index.

51. Gold and others (1996).

Those are important qualifications. Their empirical importance needs quantification.

A third reason adds to the two presented above. The QALY scale is constructed from information about preferences over different states of health. It is noted in the medical outcomes literature that the QALY is a measure of preferences, that it contains rather strong assumptions that yield something close to a measure of the economist's idea of cardinal utility.[52] Having a measure of preferences across states of health permits economists to do something in the case of health care accounting that cannot be done for automobile or computer accounting. For cars and computers, one does not have information on preferences for improvements in quality; therefore economists must find market values for them.

In summary, there are three reasons why QALY adjustments can be used directly in medical care price indexes, without the necessity for placing monetary values on them, as is necessary for quality adjustments in other goods and services. First, medical improvements are always measured in the same units. Second, incremental units are mostly attained in the future, which is already discounted in the measure. Third, the QALY measure itself has community preferences for states of health built into it. None of those conditions applies to price index quality adjustments that are available for most other goods and services. I conclude that access to QALY means that economists can incorporate improvements in medical care into price and output measures directly, without needing to put a value on life.

Some may contend, and have, that the QALY does not do what it purports to do, and these contentions are to be taken seriously. This is not the place to consider them. Rather, the present discussion concerns only a single problem: If the QALY does what it purports to do, what are the implications for using it in economic measurement?

Additionally, Mark Pauly points out (see chapter 6) that even if QALY measurements are extended and perfected, questions of accuracy remain. For medical decisionmaking, it is only necessary to determine whether the value of QALY (properly, the cost-effectiveness ratio in which QALY is the denominator) exceeds some bound. Price indexes require point estimates, which implies more accuracy. Pauly's point is correct; but the accuracy of quality adjustments for nonmedical goods

52. Ibid. It should be acknowledged, however, that this cardinal property of QALY has itself been criticized.

and services is not always high, and the choice is between using a number that is relevant (QALY) but imprecise and using no number at all.

Do Statistical Agencies Value Life Implicitly?

Statistical agency administrators have objected to price and output research in medical care that places a value on life.

The previous section showed that it may not be necessary to value life to use medical outcome measures. The present one responds to statistical agency concerns by explaining that price indexes (and therefore national accounts that use these price indexes as deflators) already value life *implicitly*.

Consider again the rows of table 7-1. Why do price index compilers only carry out comparisons within the rows? A simple answer is that moving down the columns introduces noncomparability—the content of the treatment in each row is not strictly comparable to that in another row. That answer is acceptable as far as it goes, but there is more to it.

For nonmedical goods and services, the price index literature often presents an explicit justification for restricting price comparisons to those that move across the rows of table 7-1. Any difference in price that is observed for different treatments at the same time (that is, price comparisons down the columns at the same time period or, for example, p_{b2}/p_{a2}) equals the value of the quality difference—it is a measure of willingness to pay for the more expensive treatment by those who benefit from the more expensive treatment. This presumption arises in many forms, both explicit and implicit, which need not be explored here. It justifies, for example, the common practice of "linking" across rows (bringing one treatment into the price index as a substitute for another in a way that does not change the price index, which is standard price index "matched treatment" methodology for the "new" PPI and CPI medical care indexes).

What is the medical benefit? In the case of treatments for a heart attack, it seems wholly unreasonable to contend that the benefit is not increased survival probabilities or increased life expectancy. If it is, this implies that the price-collecting agencies are implicitly assuming that price differences among medical treatments measure the value of improved life expectancy. It is true that they are seldom explicit about it. But price index procedures are implicitly valuing life whenever the differences in treatment that are controlled for in the price index (differences among the rows of table 7-1) have survival difference implications.

An alternative or analogy may be helpful. Consider an improvement in an automobile that is included in the CPI price index for automobiles. Suppose the manufacturer includes on a new model car an air-conditioning system. There is no natural way to answer the question, How much more car is this? One asks instead, What is the consumer willing to pay for this improvement? What charge is made for it? What does it sell for? What one incorporates into consumer price indexes, in general, is not a quantitative measure of the quality improvement itself but rather a quantitative measure of the value of the improvement to the user.

In medical care price indexes, the situation is a bit different. Everyone seems uncomfortable with the question, What would the consumer be willing to pay for an additional year of life? So a price index procedure—or a cost-effectiveness procedure—that *seems* to require putting an explicit monetary value on life extensions becomes controversial, essentially for ethical reasons. Yet, if another procedure values life implicitly, the same ethical reservations come into the picture. There is no reason for choosing a methodology where the ethical issue is less transparent over the one where it is more transparent.

It is true that one might engender a lively discussion about what is being bought when the more expensive treatment is chosen, and also over who is doing the choosing, but that debate applies fully to the price indexes that are currently produced. It is not unique at all to the proposals to use QALY. If someone were to contend that consumers who purchase more expensive treatments do not do so to gain medical efficacy, then the same contention destroys the entire price index logic for refusing to judge treatments A and B (or C or D) as comparable for price index purposes and for refusing to make direct price comparisons between treatments A and B (or C or D). Traditional price index methodology already requires and makes a medical efficacy assumption—that the more expensive treatment provides some medical benefit that is equal in value to the additional price charged for it.

Concluding Remarks

This chapter has developed the relation between two bodies of research—price indexes and cost-effectiveness studies—that are important in accounting for health care output and prices. Something needs to be said about the context in which that relation is of interest.

One might use effectiveness measures as quality adjustments within price indexes, national accounts, and national health accounts, as they now exist. They could be applied, that is, to the four categories of price index "quality problem" discussed above. More interesting, however, are new possibilities for health accounting that are opened up by research on medical effectiveness.

The Production Boundary in an Accounting for Health: What Expenditures Are Deflated?

Traditional national accounts (and price indexes) place a restrictive boundary on the costs that are included in economic accounting for medical care. Conventional price indexes are defined only on the charges made by medical care providers, the market transactions designated by the p_{it} and q_{it} information in table 7-1. The logic behind this restriction is apparent from equation 7-3: if a measure of output is to be formed by deflation, then the concept of "price" in the price index must match the measure of expenditure that is to be deflated. The expenditures that matter for conventional national accounts are monetary expenditures paid to medical care providers, not some wider concept of the full cost of illness or of treatment. Price indexes have been defined accordingly.

However, neither monetary expenditure nor the transaction price charged by the provider is a very good measure of the cost of illness or of the treatment of illness. Do we want to know the deflated value of expenditures on hospitals? Or do we want to compile an accounting for the total cost of illness? Of course, we want both. However, the usefulness of traditional national accounts for understanding the use of resources in health care, and for measuring health care output and productivity, is greatly limited by their restriction to market transactions.

Fortunately, broader accounts for medical costs already exist. These are sometimes called "burden-of-disease" studies. In place of the restricted concept of cost or expenditure in national accounts, the total cost of illness—direct and indirect—is estimated. This cost concept is closer to the numerator of cost-effectiveness studies than to the transactions price concept that is used in traditional national accounts.

The first government burden-of-disease study seems to be Rice's *Estimating the Cost of Illness*.[53] Subsequently, these accounts have been improved and updated several times in the United States.[54] They have also now been constructed for a number of other countries, so there are

53. Rice (1966).
54. An update to 1995 is Hodgson and Cohen (1998).

not only limited time series for some countries but also the beginning of a basis for making international comparisons of costs.

So far, burden-of-disease studies have been conducted in constant dollars. Neither the total burden estimates nor the various components that are also published have been deflated by price indexes to obtain estimates in real terms. That is the next step in improved accounting for health care.[55]

The Classifications: What Prices Do We Want to Measure?

In national accounts, and national health accounts, expenditures are classified by provider of funds and by recipient of funds. The classification tells who provides the funds (for example, the federal government) and who gets them (for example, hospitals), but it tells relatively little about what the funds are spent for.

Burden-of-disease studies classify expenditures into disease categories, not funding categories. Generally, they disaggregate to the level of ICD-9 chapters or by disease categories within ICD-9 chapters. A burden-of-disease study tells how much is spent on, say, circulatory disease or heart disease (or how much is spent with hospitals on heart disease). The burden-of-disease classification yields information that is a bit like the "product side" of conventional national accounts, which tell how much is spent on, say, consumption of restaurant meals.

The burden-of-disease classification system naturally suggests the question, What has happened to the cost of treating, for example, heart attacks or strokes? The usual national accounting classification asks instead, What has happened to the cost of hospital services? The burden-of-disease classification is a much more natural one for integrating medical outcome measures into economic accounting for health care because outcome measures are constructed for alternative treatments for a specified disease.

It is true that hospital services are made up of expenditures on diseases, so the two groupings of information are not antithetical. One could, for example, combine Cutler and others' estimates with the BLS hospital PPI for circulatory disease.[56] But "hospital services" is such a broad category; it focuses attention away from what is being treated and toward institutional groupings (type of hospital) that may be problematic

---

55. See also Triplett (1998).
56. Chapter 2.

for accounting for health care because treatment of disease too often crosses the boundaries between institutional providers. Additionally, physicians' services price indexes are not, for the most part, organized by disease, so the PPI accounting for health costs is not consistently by disease categories. Classification by disease focuses attention on the questions, What has happened to the price of treating heart attacks, on the quantity of the treatments and of their outcome? That is a more useful focus for improving our information on the real economic performance of the health care sector than is the institutional focus of the present system, with its emphasis on institutional providers of care, and on recipients of funds and the funding agencies. If adopted for economic accounts for health, the cost-of-disease focus would also have the advantage of setting up the accounts in a form that takes maximum advantage of the burgeoning research on medical outcomes and cost effectiveness.

Structuring accounts around the cost of disease has additional advantages in constructing accounts for health for countries that have public health systems. In those countries, prices charged by medical providers do not exist, at least for the bulk of medical care. A price index for the hospital industry makes no sense, nor does constructing hospital output by deflation methods. But data exist on the cost of disease and the cost of alternative treatments, on the numbers of treatments (the q_{it} terms of table 7-1), and there is growing information on medical outcomes in all countries. There is also great interest in accounting for the output and productivity of medical care in several of those countries. One can conceive of doing this by constructing direct quantity measures for health care, using medical outcome measures to "adjust" treatment quantities, instead of treatment prices. The application of that is outside the scope of this chapter.

References

Bailar, John C., III, and Heather L. Gornik. 1997. "Cancer Undefeated." *New England Journal of Medicine* 336(22): 1569–74.
Barzel, Yoram. 1969. "Productivity and the Price of Medical Services." *Journal of Political Economy* 77: 1014–27.
Bresnahan, Timothy F., and Robert J. Gordon, eds. 1997. *The Economics of New Goods.* Studies in Income and Wealth 58. University of Chicago Press.
Cardenas, Elaine. 1996. "The CPI for Hospital Services: Concepts and Procedures." *Monthly Labor Review* 119(7): 32–42.
Catron, Brian, and Bonnie Murphy. 1996. "Hospital Price Inflation: What Does the New PPI Tell Us?" *Monthly Labor Review* 120(7): 24–31.

Cutler, David M., and others. 1998. "Are Medical Prices Declining?" *Quarterly Journal of Economics* (November).

Diagnosis Related Groups Definitions Manual. 1997. Version 15.0. Wallingford, Conn.: 3M Company.

Ehrhardt, Melvin E., Raymond M. Fish, and Linda M. Tambourine. 1993. *DRG 1993: Diagnosis Related Groupings with ICD-9-CM Cross Reference.* Los Angeles: Practice Management Information Corporation.

Feldstein, Martin S. 1969. "Discussion." In *Production and Productivity in the Service Industries.* Studies in Income and Wealth 34, edited by Victor R. Fuchs. Columbia University Press

Fuchs, Victor R., ed. 1969. *Production and Productivity in the Service Industries.* Studies in Income and Wealth 34. Columbia University Press.

Garber, Alan M., and Charles E. Phelps. 1997. "Economic Foundations of Cost-Effectiveness Analysis." *Journal of Health Economics* 16: 1–31.

Gold, Marthe R., and others, eds. 1996. *Cost-Effectiveness in Health and Medicine.* New York: Oxford University Press.

Griliches, Zvi, ed. 1971. *Price Indexes and Quality Change: Studies in New Methods of Measurement.* Harvard University Press.

———. 1992. *Output Measurement in the Service Sectors.* Studies in Income and Wealth 56. University of Chicago Press.

Hodgson, Thomas A., and Alan J. Cohen. 1998. "Medical Care Expenditures for Major Diseases, 1995." National Center for Health Statistics, Centers for Disease Control and Prevention.

Lazenby, Helen C., and others. 1992. "National Health Accounts: Lessons from the U.S. Experience." *Health Care Financing Review* 13(4): 89–103.

Meltzer, David. 1997. "Accounting for Future Costs in Medical Cost-Effectiveness Analysis." *Journal of Health Economics* 16:33–64.

Moulton, Brent R., and Karin E. Moses. 1997. "Addressing the Quality Change Issue in the Consumer Price Index." *Brookings Papers on Economic Activity* 1: 305–49.

Murray, Christopher J. L., and Alan D. Lopez, eds. 1996. *Global Burden of Disease: A Comprehensive Assessment of Mortality and Disability from Diseases, Injuries, and Risk Factors in 1990 and Projected to 2020.* 2 vols. Harvard University Press.

Newhouse, Joseph P. 1989. "Measuring Medical Prices and Understanding Their Effects: The Baxter Prize Address." *Journal of Health Administration Education* 7(1): 19–26.

Phelps, Charles E., and Alvin I. Mushlin. 1991. "On the (Near) Equivalence of Cost-Effectiveness and Cost-Benefit Analyses." *International Journal of Technology Assessment in Health Care* 7(1): 12–21.

Puckett, Craig D., ed. 1997. *1997 Annual Hospital Version, the Educational Annotation of ICD-9-CM.* 5th ed. 3 vols. Reno: Channel.

Reder, M. W. 1969. "Some Problems in the Measurement of Productivity in the Medical Care Industry." In *Production and Productivity in the Service Industries.* Studies in Income and Wealth 34, edited by Victor R. Fuchs. Columbia University Press

Rice, Dorothy P. 1966. *Estimating the Cost of Illness.* Health Economics Series 6. Government Printing Office.

Rice, Dorothy P., and Loucele A. Horowitz. 1967. "Trends in Medical Care Prices." *Social Security Bulletin* 30(7): 13–28.

Schelling, T. C. 1968. "The Life You Save May Be Your Own." *Problems in Public Expenditure Analysis*. Studies of Government Finance. Brookings Institution.

Scitovsky, Anne A. 1964. "An Index of the Cost of Medical Care: A Proposed New Approach." In *The Economics of Health and Medical Care*. 1st Conference on the Economics of Health and Medical Care, University of Michigan, 1962. University of Michigan.

———. 1967. "Changes in the Costs of Treatment of Selected Illnesses, 1951–65." *American Economic Review* 57(5): 1182–95.

Triplett, Jack E. 1989. "Price and Technological Change in a Capital Good: A Survey of Research on Computers." In *Technology and Capital Formation*, edited by Dale W. Jorgenson and Ralph Landau. MIT Press.

———. 1997. "Measuring Consumption: The Post-1973 Slowdown and the Research Issues." *Review: Federal Reserve Bank of St. Louis* 79(3): 9–42.

———. 1998. "What's Different about Health? Human Repair and Car Repair in National Accounts." Paper presented at the Conference on Research in Income and Wealth's "Conference on Medical Care," Bethesda, Md., June 12–13, 1998.

U.S. Congress. Joint Economic Committee, Subcommittee on Economic Statistics. 1961. *Government Price Statistics: Hearings before the Subcommittee on Economic Statistics of the Joint Economic Committee*, 87 Cong., 1 sess., May 1, 2, 3, 4, and 5, part 2.

U.S. Department of Commerce. Economics and Statistics Administration and Bureau of Economic Analysis. 1996. *Survey of Current Business* 76 (1–2).

Weinstein, Milton C., and Willard G. Manning, Jr. 1997. "Theoretical Issues in Cost-Effectiveness Analysis." *Journal of Health Economics* 16: 121–28.

8

Health Care Prices, Outcomes, and Policy

Outcomes from the Viewpoint of a Federal Agency
John M. Eisenberg

THE AGENCY FOR Health Care Policy and Research (AHCPR) was established in 1989 as part of the same legislation that created the resource-based relative value scale for physician payment. As Congress sought to rationalize physician payment, it also concluded that the nation needed better information about the outcomes and effectiveness of medical care. Clinicians and patients needed better information on outcomes to make decisions that would use health care resources most effectively. Soon after its establishment, AHCPR became the "outcomes agency" and helped foster a boom in outcomes research in this country.

The agency, in its first eight years, has sponsored outcomes research, including $100 million on twenty-five Patient Outcome Research Teams, of which eleven were in progress in 1997. AHCPR also sponsored the development of a set of practice guidelines that got the agency in a bit of political hot water but also established a scientific and impartial standard for the design of practice guidelines that others have emulated.

Although AHCPR is a new agency, the challenge of using evidence of effectiveness to improve medical care is a very old topic. In fact, Florence Nightingale is said to have commented in 1863, "I am feign to sum up with an urgent appeal for adopting this or some other uniform system of publishing the statistical records of hospitals. If they could be obtained, they would show subscribers how their money was being spent, what amount of good was really being done with it and whether the money was doing mischief rather than good."

I regret to report to you that, 134 years later, we still aspire to meet Nightingale's challenge. We still are trying to find out whether more mischief or good is being done with the services our hospitals offer their patients. Today I want to set a framework for outcomes research, that is, for understanding the end results of clinical services, the denominator of the cost-effectiveness ratio, and the outcomes of medical care.

A Continuum of Outcomes Measures

There is a continuum of outcomes measures that can be used to describe the effectiveness of medical care. These range from traditional clinical outcomes, such as mortality or whether a disease has been cured, to physiologic measures that are surrogates for clinical outcomes. These physiologic measures of outcomes include indicators such as electro-cardiographic or cardiac enzyme changes for patients who might have had a myocardial infarction (heart attack) or blood pressure changes for patients whose hypertension threatens to cause damage to their hearts, kidneys, or brains. Changes in the millimeters of mercury of blood pressure may not be a very useful outcome in the short term for how people feel, but clinical research shows no doubt about the relationship between blood pressure levels and long-term outcomes.

In addition to traditional clinical measures, such as mortality and cure rates, and in addition to physiologic measures, a third outcomes measure is clinical events, such as myocardial infarctions. For example, a cost-effectiveness analysis using this measure of outcome might be reported in dollars per myocardial infarction averted. A fourth is people's perceptions of their health, or their symptoms, for example, the amount of angina (chest pain from coronary disease) a patient suffers, as measured perhaps by a symptom score for angina. However, when we move beyond these clinical outcomes, which are the results that have been used traditionally in clinical research and in clinical practice, to measure patient-reported outcomes, we struggle to identify measures that accurately reflect how patients feel about the results they experience. The added dimension of outcomes research has been the development of measures that reflect patients' values and preferences for their health states.

As we move up the ladder of outcomes measures, we find the need to develop better measures that reflect not only physiologic changes but also changes in how people feel. There are increasingly well-validated functional measures that describe how well people are able to carry out important activities, and there are now preference measures that address more of the issues that economists find attractive, especially those based on patients' perceived and measured utilities, or their values for these health states.

One of the challenges that we face in the outcomes research field is distinguishing the optimal use of general and disease-specific outcomes. The comment was made at the "Measuring the Prices of Medical Treatments" conference about how difficult it is to aggregate outcomes across diseases. In part, that is because the general outcomes that are often used are so general that any differences that may occur among different clinical interventions are too narrow to make a difference in general functioning, even if they are important for one aspect of patients' health states. However, these differences may make a substantial difference when we measure disease-specific functional status.

For example, a difference in how well a drug treats my skin rash may be measurable but may be too narrow a health outcome to affect how I feel about my overall health. Conversely, the Short Form 36 is a classic and widely accepted general functional measure. But this general measure may not detect changes in one aspect of health. AHCPR has a number of projects that have developed new ways of measuring outcomes that address this issue. A project at Massachusetts General Hospital and Dartmouth developed a BPH (benign prostatic hypertrophy) symptom-problem index, a measure of health status specifically directed at the changes that occur as a result of enlargement of the prostate gland, such as concerns about urination. We were pleased to learn that the article describing this work is now one of the most frequently quoted articles in the urologic literature. This research demonstrates that this new form of health care scholarship—outcomes research—is becoming a part of the lexicon of clinicians who are doing clinical research.

Other outcome measures address the broader question of patients' satisfaction. One new measure that we have developed at AHCPR is the Consumer Assessment of Health Plans Survey, which is increasingly being adopted as a measure of patients' experience with the care they receive. We know from multiple studies that satisfaction with care is linked with both disease-specific and general outcomes.

Uses of Outcomes Measures

These new measures of outcomes can be used as the denominator in cost-effectiveness analysis and increasingly are becoming a key element in the evaluation of health care services and technology. There are, of course, many uses of outcome measures other than cost-effectiveness analysis. One that will get attention from the President's Advisory Commission on Consumer Protection and Quality in the Health Care Industry is the degree to which we can use these outcome measures as an indicator of the quality of health care. Better measures and better reporting of outcomes can inform consumers who are making choices about plans or providers and who want to know more about the quality or the outcomes they can expect. Better measures of outcomes can also help plans and providers identify opportunities for quality improvement, that is, to help those who provide care learn what their patients' outcomes are so that they can improve them.

Another use for outcomes research is to measure the results of clinical trials. AHCPR has been pleased that the National Institute of Health's clinical trials are increasingly using more sophisticated outcome measures and adopting some of the measures that have been developed by AHCPR and its investigators. Clinical practice guidelines and recommendations are another use for outcomes defined and measured through careful research.

Researchers also are investigating population-based measures of outcomes as an assessment of the health status of populations. This is still another attractive use of outcomes measures, that is, to understand the health of the public.

Some Challenges

Case mix and severity adjustment are important issues in the use of outcome measures in health care. It is difficult to use outcomes to assess the quality of care unless we can adjust the results to the severity of the patient's condition and other factors that may affect their health, even including social and economic factors. We also need to understand better how different cultural groups value health outcomes differently, because if we aggregate outcomes across populations, we may blunt not only individual preferences but also differences among ethnic and cultural groups, which may advantage or disadvantage some.

Finally, it will be important to continue to develop links between intermediate outcomes, some of those that are easily measured like millimeters of mercury reduction in blood pressure, to intermediate outcomes, like reductions in myocardial infarction or stroke, and to ultimate outcomes, the measures of preference and utility-based health status.

The study of outcomes—and their use as a denominator of cost-effectiveness ratios as well as other uses—offers the nation a challenging research agenda and one that we hope to foster at AHCPR. Broader use of outcomes measures in all aspects of health care delivery can help us understand and achieve excellence in medical care.

The Future of Health Care Policy
Willard G. Manning Jr.

L IKE MARK PAULY, I am not someone who has done an awful lot with index number problems. Nevertheless, I found interesting the discussion of the underlying issues that we need for making welfare comparisons. A number of diligent efforts have been made by individuals to try to understand the process by which we move from one place to another, which things should be counted, how they should be counted. I think there is recognition that simply keeping track of the inputs in the way that was traditionally done was inappropriate and becoming more inappropriate.

As Jack Triplett and Dennis Fixler have described in this volume, the Bureau of Labor Statistics is moving to measure price change on a treatment basis. I think a movement in this direction is to be desired because it is a lot closer to what it is that we are ultimately interested in. However, I think we should move, ideally, to what we would like to measure. In essence, what we are trying to do is to find out something about what it costs to produce survival and quality of life (whether you use that term in the sense that cost-effectiveness analysis uses it or not), as the technologies change, and as we have opportunities to live longer or better lives than we did before. I do not know whether that is practical.

What we have seen in chapters 2 and 3 are attempts to take two quite different situations and go through that exercise: trace the linkage between the production process and some measure of the thing that the customers, clients, or patients (whatever you want to call them) actually value—increases in health status, functioning, or survival.

To the extent that this enterprise (that is, research on price index measurement) leads in that direction, I hope that we will be able to take the next step, going beyond doing it on a treatment basis. The treatments themselves are not constant; they change over time, disappear in ways that Jack Triplett has laid out in chapter 7, and new ones are developed. But we could, in principle, think of people having stable preferences for various attributes, such as the quality of their lives, or life expectancy, or survival. The current technology is just one way of getting these attributes, and different technologies provide different costs at the margin as we go through time. We do not have to worry so much about things coming and going as we do whether people actually value treatment per se. People do not value treatment per se, except for a limited number of cases.

Having two chapters that are as different in the illnesses they discuss as those two chapters highlights some of what we need to learn about this price analysis: understanding the production process and what goes into the valuation decision. In addition, I think we need to go through these studies because in the process of performing a number of these exercises, we will learn a great deal about what the issues are, what the difficulties are, and what the analytic problems are that we are going to have to deal with. It may seem that doing everything by three- or four-digit ICD-9 codes is an impossible task, let alone pulling in the CPT manual and going through it. But I think we could, in fact, learn a lot from these kinds of exercises.

I would however, encourage much of the work, if possible, to go back to the old Gary Becker–Kelvin Lancaster kind of view of the world, or the health production process, the Michael Grossman approach.[1] Some of what was then an interesting way of telling a story may have more practical implications now. It may be more doable than it once was, and it also may keep us on track in terms of measuring some of the right things.

The other comments I want to make have to do with cost-effectiveness analysis. Before I continue, I want to make it clear that I am not trying to be an apologist for cost-effectiveness analysis (or CEA) per se, but I think that we have to realize that cost-effectiveness analysis does try to do something fundamentally different in some respects from the welfare comparisons that are embedded in cost-of-living adjustments or price indexes.

I think in some communities, such as health, there is a fundamental unwillingness to buy into willingness to pay at the individual level—not so much because it measures preferences as a concern about whether it really measures ability to pay, a distinction that economists usually forget. So what is attempted in cost-effectiveness analysis is to measure the quality-adjusted life-year, or QALY. This appeals to a lot of people because they see it as a way of avoiding ability to pay. Then they can pick a threshold of cost per QALY and use that as a decision rule that, from a societal point of view, is equitable. We do not give treatment to Bill Gates just because Bill Gates is rich enough to afford it and deny it to somebody else because they are not.

1. Becker (1965); Lancaster (1966); Grossman (1972).

The almost equivalence of CEA and CBA (cost-benefit analysis) is just that: almost equivalent, but not exactly. For that reason, I think we have to keep in mind that CEA has been used for making what are basically egalitarian and distributional modifications to an allocation system. The modifications may not be truly appropriate when you think of what belongs in a true price index. A true price index is the ratio between what you would have to spend to get the old level of utility at the current prices relative to what you actually paid out in the old period. It buys into the existing income distribution, the difference in tastes and in the ability to pay.

The cost-of-living index is answering a different question and uses different input data. Crossing back and forth between this index and CEA ignores the fact that they have two quite different purposes. Many of the problems with CEA arise from this desire to get at an egalitarian decision. As a result, CEA makes a lot of what we would consider errors. Mark Pauly does a nice job, I think, of laying out some of those (see chapter 6), such as the omission of aspects of risk aversion and the failure—my particular hobbyhorse—to think that all QALYs could be different. For example, if you have a group that is at high risk, it is both egalitarian and more efficient from a Pareto sense to give more resources to the high-risk group for a given reduction in mortality risk. But that is something that is not captured in cost effectiveness.

In substance, CEA is not quite egalitarian and, needless to say, not quite efficient. So a number of issues come up in cost-effectiveness analysis that we need to keep in mind. CEA differs in its recommendation for using community preferences rather than individual preferences.[2] The community's preferences do not matter, except in certain circumstances, for doing a cost-of-living index or price index. What matters are the preferences of the people who actually use the service. If it is treatment for angina, somebody's dread of angina and heart disease is not a factor if it does not apply to them, but would matter for people who are suffering from angina.

The last issue that comes up about cost-effectiveness analysis is the recommendations as to which costs get captured. I think, actually, what was proposed by Gold and others is probably more correct than what is conventionally done in the cost-of-living literature.[3] Our recommendations on calculating the incremental cost included evaluation of the inputs that were not a part of monetary transactions but are directly related to treatment.[4] So if you do not decide to put your mother or your father in

2. Going back to Gold and others (1996).
3. By myself as well.
4. Gold and others (1996).

a nursing home but instead take him into your own home, and you or your wife partially drop out of the labor force in order to provide that care, the cost-effectiveness analysis should consider alternative modalities for taking care of somebody with those conditions, and would account for the opportunity cost associated with that time.

Traditionally in price indexes and national accounts, because of the production boundary, this is not the case. For all intents and purposes, from the point of view of the usual calculation of the cost-of-living index, anybody's time provided without a transaction is worth nothing. But I think that if we go back to the conceptual basis for the cost-of-living index, at least in economic theory, what we want to do is make this welfare comparison that is based on differences in opportunity costs. If I have to make a labor-or-leisure choice, or my wife has to make this choice, some things get taken out of the formal marketplace but get done in kind.

Now, there are all sorts of reasons for not including those nonmarket costs in a variety of analyses. In a lot of cost-effectiveness analyses, if you change the perspective to being the employers or being the insurance plans, many of these nonmarket issues also go away. Maybe there is an equivalent justification for the national accounts production boundary. In a very real sense, if we have a world in which activities are going across major boundaries over time—if people are paying to go out to dinner because they both work now, if they are paying for laundry services and such—then any analysis that ignores in-kind provision of those services or household production, in fact, leads to a biased estimate of the welfare changes associated with shifts over time. That is an issue I wanted to raise about the construction of cost-of-living indexes and accounting for health, because it may be a substantial element in the calculation of the true cost of living.

The Shape of Health Care Research
David Meltzer

WILL MANNING REMINDED us earlier of Oscar Wilde's comment that an economist is someone who knows the price of everything and the value of nothing. As I reflect on some of my physician colleagues, I realize that one could similarly joke that doctors are people who know the price of nothing and think they

know the value of everything. I hope that I, as a physician and an economist, will get the better of those combinations, as opposed to the worst.

Two fundamental questions are addressed by most of the chapters
here. First, do the changes in health care expenditures reflect rising prices
or increasing quality or quantity? The basic insight here is that changes
in quality that are not measured can appear in changes in price and can
overstate the true price change. Of course, the opposite holds when
quality is falling, as may be the case for treatment of depression in the
United States.

The second question is whether these expenditures are worth it. I think
the key to both of these questions is the more basic question of what is the
value of health care, and how do we measure it. I think it is worthwhile,
even at this late hour, to go back to some very basic questions of microeconomics to remind ourselves what question we are asking ourselves.

The simple consumer problem says that consumer welfare is maxi-
mized when consumers are able to choose their expenditures, subject to
the budget constraint, to maximize utility. If you can figure out how a
change in prices or income affects the level of utility that is achieved, you
can determine how it has affected welfare. Well, in the real world, we do
not have the luxury of seeing indifference curves or having ways to
directly observe information about preferences that could be used to
analyze the welfare impacts of price changes.

Instead, when prices change, all we really observe are shifts in the
choices people make. Economic theory actually tells us very little. It tells
us that if you get more of everything, you are better off. It tells us if you
end up with something you could have had before, but did not choose,
you are worse off, or if you end up choosing something new when you
could have had what you previously had, you are better off. That is
revealed preference. When other shifts occur in which you end up with
more of one commodity and less of the other, economic theory alone
does not tell us anything. Can we figure out what it is people value? Can
we understand the structure of their preferences?

This issue is implicitly dealt with in every one of these chapters. The
Cutler study says that happiness is living, avoiding mortality. Following
this approach, we do not worry about quality of life. The Frank, Berndt
and Busch chapter deals with the issue by saying something about the
production function for health. Do you meet the guideline for care of
depression? The price indexes they talk about are really statements about
the curvature of this indifference curve. Likewise, the Ellison and Hellerstein chapter really does the same thing, as does the Pauly chapter, which

suggests asking how much are you willing to pay for one thing as opposed to another? In chapter 7, Jack Triplett talks about the QALY concept and raises the same issues.

In fact, in the case of health care, it is more complicated than this. We have both an indifference curve and a health production function that are embedded together. So, the lesson of all of these chapters is that the key question is: How do we value health care? That is the key to understanding whether people are better off. That is the key to constructing price indexes. So, if we can answer this question, we can in fact answer those two questions we came here to try to answer today.

One important issue is the right level of aggregation. How should we define the goods for which we want to determine price? We have seen many different ways of thinking about this over time. In the very earliest price indexes, people thought about a very narrowly defined good: What is the price of a hospital day? Or, what is the price of a colonoscopy?

Alternatively, you can think in broader groups. What is the price of finding colon cancer? What is the price of cancer diagnosis and treatment? What is the price, perhaps, of insurance? That is what Mark Pauly has suggested. You can think more broadly still: What is the cost of saving a year of life? Or, even, what is the price of saving a quality-adjusted life-year? These are the broader scopes to think about. It is a difficult choice. The more narrowly you define the question, the easier it is to figure out whether the price is actually rising. But the answer may also be less relevant.

Do we really care if the price of a colonoscopy is rising if, in fact, we can find tumors by a stool guaiac, which is an alternative diagnostic approach for colon cancer? I think the answer is we probably do not care.

So why do we even care about price indexes for health care? It seems to me this depends on how we are going to use them, and this question has not been adequately addressed here. Addressing those issues would help us move this discussion forward in very important ways.

Which one of these multiple measures should you use? At what level should you aggregate? I think the answer depends a lot on how you intend to use the measure. If you just want to know whether the price of some narrowly defined good is rising for whatever reason, perhaps reflecting a shift in supply, then, just measure the price of that very narrow good. On the other hand, if you want to understand whether the value of health care is increasing, you must aggregate and look at other things.

The techniques that we use to answer these questions will reflect how we ultimately intend to use the information. If we just want to know whether the price of a colonoscopy is rising, we would be looking for a needle in a haystack by examining the differences in growth of the price of insurance plans that include and exclude colonoscopy, even if we could find them.

On the other hand, if we want to know what the value of health care is, we would be crazy to try to price out colonoscopies, price out beta-blockers, price out everything, and then try to add them together. The only way to do that, in fact, is to know, in addition, the structure of the indifference curve. As difficult as that question is, it is, in a lot of ways, unavoidable if you want to answer this correctly.

How should we be trying to understand the shape of this utility function, that is, people's relative value of different health expenditures? I think the big competition here—and it's a competition truly of weaklings—is between the willingness-to-pay and quality-adjusted life-year approaches. Mark Pauly clearly says what he has argued forcefully in the past, that willingness-to-pay makes a lot more sense. Jack Triplett gives a little more emphasis to the QALY approach.

I should point out that the willingness-to-pay approach, despite its guise of being somehow more theoretically sound, in fact, is not perfect. Because I am willing to pay more for something than you are, we decide that we should do what I want; however, if I do not pay you for it, you are not better off. The connection between willingness-to-pay and welfare economics is not perfect.

But the bigger problems are the empirical problems. Mark Pauly has talked a little bit about some of the problems with willingness-to-pay. People will pay $5 to preserve some species they have never heard of. They will pay $5 for a whole group of species, just the same way. This is the problem of aggregation in environmental economics.

Likewise, QALYs have many problems. There are face validity problems with QALYs. There are questions about how people deal with risk. And the problems go on and on. But I think Mark actually brought up the key test, and this is what I want to emphasize. In fact, there is a gold standard out there, and I think that is what we need to work toward. Even though you might think we do not have one, I think we have something that is not far from a gold standard, and that is the way that we make almost all decisions in society: we inform people about choices, and we let them choose. It is actual behavior. What we need to ask ourselves is whether we can find a gold standard of value and then see how these measures line up to it.

The standard of a valid measure of value is whether it predicts behavior. We can apply this standard and let these proposals for measuring value compete against each other. In other words, what does a better job of predicting what people actually do when they have a choice? Does the willingness-to-pay approach do a better job? Or does the QALY approach do a better job? And, in fact, the interesting thing is we already have some evidence about that.

Let me show you two studies and contrast these things. One is a study contrasting a willingness-to-pay approach to the valuation of strawberries to an actual series of purchases made. In fact, they lined up almost exactly.[5]

Now, we also have some studies on QALYs. There is one single study that looks at this, comparing treatments for benign prostatic hypertrophy.[6] The study asked people various QALY questions and then figured out which treatment generated the most QALYs for a patient. Medical treatment for your benign prostatic hypertrophy or surgical treatment, which gives you the bigger gain in QALYs, in quality-adjusted life-years? What they found was that QALYs did an excellent job of sorting the surgical patients and the medical patients. Patients who chose surgery were in fact the patients calculated to have the bigger gain in QALYs from surgery.

The major criticism of this study is that these were questions asked of people after they had already made their decision, so this is probably self-justifying behavior: people answering to minimize cognitive dissonance. I am doing some work now in which I try to address this question in a more prospective manner, looking at patients' decisions about adopting intensive therapy for diabetes.[7] What I am finding is that QALYs do not do as well as this, but they do have some ability to predict choices. And, of course, strawberries are not the same thing as health, so we can hardly assume that willingness-to-pay will predict health behaviors. We have a lot to learn.

Measuring Health Care Prices: What Research Is Needed?
Burton A. Weisbrod

WHAT KINDS OF research are needed on price measurement in the health sector? These comments are intended not as criticism of current measurement techniques but as potential guides for research on what should be measured and how.

5. Brookshire, Coursey, and Schulze (1987).
6. Krumins, Fihn, and Kent (1988).
7. Meltzer and Polonsky (1998).

Price Changes as Welfare Measures

The first requirement is to be clear about what we want to measure. I suggest that our goal should be to measure the change in "welfare" resulting from a change in "price." That is, the fundamental theoretic perspective is that price indexes should be thought of as indexes of welfare: other factors equal, a change in price reflects a change in welfare in the opposite direction. However, whether it is reasonable to assume that other welfare-affecting variables will remain constant as some price changes is a matter deserving attention.

The difficulty of measuring prices when quality is changing is well known. One aspect of that difficulty that has not received attention is the effect of increased knowledge on consumers' assessment and valuation of some product, even when the physical commodity has not changed at all. As scientific knowledge expands we often learn about new, or newly important, attributes of a commodity that cause us to evaluate the commodity as having changed in quality even though it is only our knowledge of it that has changed. For example, a quart of whole milk today may be identical to the milk sold "yesterday," but "quality" may not be constant in the sense that Bovine Growth Hormone is recognized today, but was not recognized previously, as a relevant dimension of quality. A good may be of constant physical quality but of changed quality in the welfare sense. "Quality" is more complex than is traditionally recognized.

The Commodity to Be Priced

What is the commodity for which price changes should be observed? Mark Pauly has suggested (chapter 6) that in health care we should be measuring the prices not of health services but of health care *insurance*. This deserves attention, although it seems likely that the correlation will be high between the prices of insurance and those of the underlying services. It is true, however, that, even granted that the "price" of an insurance contract is a function of the prices of the services insured against, it is also a function of the expected quantities of those services. Thus the price of an insurance contract that covers a given set of health care services is a function of quantities, whereas price indexes generally attempt to abstract from changes in quantities.

Another issue relevant to the use of health care insurance as the unit of service to be priced is, once again, the measurement of changes in quality. Even if the wording of an insurance policy is unchanged over time, technological advances change the set of services covered, and it would be a strong assumption that quality of care is unaffected; thus an unchanged premium for insurance does not reflect unchanged welfare if the quality of services covered by the insurance has improved.

It is noteworthy, as we think about the constancy of quality of a commodity over time, that health insurance contracts are not available now with coverage limited to services that were available at some prior time. Such a contract, were it available, would permit pricing of a constant set of services. It would not deal, however, with the quality improvements available under other insurance contracts, of the types generally available today. Why such constant-technology insurance contracts are not available is a matter deserving study, in part because of the implications for welfare measurement. That is, the unavailability may reflect the absence of demand, which would, in turn, imply that welfare is increased by purchasing increased quality.

The implications of redefining what to price for measurement purposes—from specific health services, or even from treating a specified illness—deserve further study and assessment. The diffusion of new health care technologies is not instantaneous, and it varies considerably by geographic region. This suggests that there is what amounts to a natural experiment occurring in response to technological advances. There is information content from that "experiment." We should seek to understand how to interpret the differential diffusion rates for new technologies as reflections of their social value. This, in turn, can aid measurement of the real price of health care.

Welfare and Willingness to Pay for Health Care

Interpreting consumers' willingness to pay for health care as a measure of welfare is complex. It is clear, as the growing literature on "contingent valuation" indicates, that sophisticated methods of eliciting such information are being developed. It is also the case, however, that when health care involves services and situations with which consumers have little or no experience, they may not be able to provide meaningful estimates of willingness to pay. More fundamentally, however, there is a question of whether resource allocation to medical care *should* be based on willingness to pay, assuming that it can be determined. It is arguable that society judges that the existing income distribution, while ethically acceptable for determining the distribution of most outputs, should not determine access to health care. In this sense individuals' willingness to pay for their own health care is not relevant or, at least, is not the sole determinant of efficient resource allocation. Society may hold the ethical position that increased length of life is a fundamentally different commodity from, say, a chocolate cookie. However, such a social judgment could be interpreted as reflecting a willingness of some people to pay to provide health care to others, and that might be discernible from willingness-to-pay measures.

Relatedly, willingness to pay is meaningful only within a particular system of property rights, and in the health care sector there are ambiguities about those rights. An illustration involving an admittedly extreme situation can help make the point: Consider a mountain climber who breaks her leg at the top of a mountain. What is the concept of willingness to pay that is relevant to the measurement of the "value" of providing health services, in the form of a rescue operation, to this disabled person? Is it the sum that the climber is willing to *pay* to be rescued? That sum reflects, of course, the person's wealth, which limits what could be paid. Or is the relevant concept the sum that the climber would have to *be paid* to forgo the rescue? That is not limited by the person's wealth, so it can be enormously greater. The difference between the two measures of the value of this health care service—the rescue—is a reflection of differential property rights—in this case, whether the individual does or does not have the "right" to the particular service.

"Costs": Which Costs and Whose Should Be Measured?

Discussions of costs of health services—in the context of measurement of prices—often fail to deal with fundamental issues of precisely which costs should be included. "Cost" is ambiguous. Typically what is measured as the cost or price of some medical care input is not its *social* cost but the *private* cost to some particular party. Consider, for example, a new health care technology that is receiving growing attention—telemedicine, a generic term for the marriage of computer and video technologies. Its cost is being studied by the Health Care Financing Administration in an attempt to establish Medicare policy. Emphasis, however, is on measuring *budgetary* costs that would be incurred by the government if this class of technologies were covered by Medicare. Potentially large savings that could be achieved for patients, in the form of reduced travel time and expense made possible by remote diagnostic and treatment applications, are unlikely to be counted since they are not covered by insurance under existing law.

A similar distinction between policies that reduce social costs and those that reduce costs to a particular provider group involves efforts to cut "costs" by reducing prices (wages) of health care input providers. When HMOs or other insurers exert monopsony power to force down hospital prices, for example, health care budgetary costs to the insurer may decline, but that might well mean that there has been a redistribution of income—from input suppliers, such as nurses, to insurers or patients. Such a redistribution may or may not be judged to be desirable. Terming it, however, a *cost reduction*, confuses real efficiency gains with income transfers.

The magnitudes and implications of systematic differences between social costs and government (or private insurer) budgetary costs deserves greater attention from the research community. Incentives to optimize budgetary costs, rather than real social costs, can be expected to distort behavior.

References

Becker, Gary S. 1965. "A Theory of the Allocation of Time." *Economic Journal* 75 (September): 493–517.

Brookshire, David S., Don L. Coursey, and William D. Schulze. 1987. "The External Validity of Experimental Economics Techniques: Analysis of Demand Behavior." *Economic Inquiry* 25(2) (April): 239–50.

Gold, Marthe R., and others, eds. 1996. *Cost-Effectiveness in Health and Medicine.* New York: Oxford University Press.

Grossman, Michael. 1972. *The Demand for Health: A Theoretical and Empirical Investigation.* New York: Columbia University Press for the National Bureau of Economic Research.

Krumins, P., S. Fihn, and D. Kent. 1988. "Symptom Severity and Patient's Values in the Decision to Perform a Transurethral Resection of the Prostate." *Medical Decision Making* 8(1): 1–8.

Lancaster, Kelvin J. 1966. "A New Approach to Consumer Theory." *Journal of Political Economy* 74 (April): 132–57.

Meltzer, David, and Tamar Polonsky. 1998. "Do Quality-Adjusted Life Years Reflect Patient Preferences? Validation Using Revealed Preference for Intensive Treatment of Insulin-Dependent Diabetes Mellitus." *Medical Decision Making* 18 (October): 459.

Contributors

Ernst R. Berndt
Massachusetts Institute of Technology

Susan H. Busch
Harvard University

Thomas W. Croghan
Eli Lilly Company

David Cutler
Harvard University

Patricia M. Danzon
University of Pennsylvania

John M. Eisenberg
Agency for Health Care Policy and Research

Sara Fisher Ellison
Massachusetts Institute of Technology

Dennis Fixler
Bureau of Labor Statistics

Richard G. Frank
Harvard University

Henry Grabowski
Duke University

Joel W. Hay
University of Southern California

Judith K. Hellerstein
University of Maryland

Willard G. Manning Jr.
University of Chicago

Mark McClellan
Stanford University

David Meltzer
University of Chicago

Joseph Newhouse
Harvard University

Mark V. Pauly
University of Pennsylvania

Charles E. Phelps
University of Rochester

Jack E. Triplett
Brookings Institution

Burton A. Weisbrod
Northwestern University

Winnie Yu
University of Pittsburgh

Index